HOW TO GET INTO MEDICAL SCHOOL

It's a Battle and Here's the Winning Strategy

Ann Twum, DPM
Arlene Blake McCain, MD

Kisslim Publishing

This book is dedicated to the bright, eager, empathetic minds who genuinely love helping and healing living beings.
To our Aunt Evelyn, a retired registered nurse who succumbed to Covid-19. She was one of the progenitors of our medical careers. May she Rest in Peace.

To my mom who unknowingly cemented this wonderful career in my mind as a done deal.
To Kam, Kris and Dre, my heartbeats and inspiration. To the next generation of doctors in the family.
AT

I also dedicate this book to my parents Segree and Faye who started the fire, my husband Trevor McCain who grabbed the fire ball and encouraged it, my siblings Heather Blake and Dr. Kurt Blake who keep the love flowing to fan the flames and, to my Daughter Rachael M. T. McCain who keeps the drive to make the fire ball as huge as the sun hoping this piece begins to light up the world.
ABM

CONTENTS

INTRODUCTION

Dr. Ann:

It was a beautiful, sunny, spring day in New York City. I opened the front door of our Brooklyn home and there was the mail. I picked up the pile mindlessly and threw it inside, lingering to admire the flowers, bask in the sun a little and breathe in the pollen filled air which I would pay for later. I came back inside, sorted through the mail and there it was - a letter from the New York College of Podiatric Medicine. My heart skipped a beat it seemed. I had forgotten, crazy as it may seem, that I had completed my application to this one school and had gotten an interview. I was busy enjoying the last semester of college where the courses were easy and unnecessary or so we seniors thought. I quickly opened the letter, read the first line and immediately saw the life of which I had dreamed flash before me as a reality. I had been accepted! I was going to be a doctor! I screamed but no one was at home to hear it. It was a regular weekday, and I was on my way to classes on campus. I called my mom to give her the good news, knowing that she would fill in everyone. I silently screamed with joy and floated through the rest of the day. I floated the ten-block walk to the subway, I floated to Dr. K's lab and then to Dr. C's lab to thank them for their letters of recommendation. I floated to my advisor's office to thank her for everything. That day was one of the best days of my life and I will never forget that joyous feeling- I was going to be a doctor!

Since then, we have 3 medical doctors in the family, an Ivy League trained scientist, one podiatrist, a veterinary medical student and a brand-new medical student. I think we just all had a love for STEM and our love for medicine grew from there. My cousin, the mother of two medical doctors, insists that neither she nor her husband pushed their children into medicine. The children confirm this. It was a passion that formed at a young age. Then came the encouragement and support. We all had different pathways- some started medical school as early as 19 years old and another in his late 40's. Studying hard was a habit and a privilege for us. Arlene was known to be incommunicado for weeks at a time when she would study for exams! However, the non-academic requirements for medical school would prove to be a bit of a challenge for some of us. Hence the interest in writing this book. **We will share with you the strategies we used that worked for our family and others.**

So, you want to be a medical doctor too. It is one of the most altruistic, selfless and humbling careers that you have chosen to pursue. It says a lot about you- the desire to help and heal people. However, getting into medical school can be a difficult task and the acceptance statistics are brutally low. The overall acceptance rate is 46%. However, if you have your heart set on attending a particular school, the acceptance rate drops to 1%-5%. The American Association of Medical Colleges (AAMC) says this about students who want to go to medical school: '**100,000 start the process, but only 50,000 complete it**. Of the roughly 100,000 applications that are started, only about 51,000 are completed each year. There are a number of reasons why an applicant may not compete an application.' I would go further: The one statistic that is unknown is the number of students who start on the premed track with intentions of going to medical school but drop out of their college's premed program because they have no support or guidance. They don't even make it to the application stage!

The good news is that there is a proven strategy that will set you apart from the **56,000** other students that will apply to medical school this year. And, yea, they all have great GPAs and MCAT scores too. These strategies apply to Veterinary medical school, Dental school, Podiatric medical school and Physician Assistant school.

It's a battle! Join us as we lay out a winning strategy for you in the chapters of this book. **By the time you complete this book you will have a solid plan of action to get accepted into medical school**.

This book was born out of the frustration from watching brilliant, hard-working relatives and friends trying to gain acceptance to medical school or having the desire to do so without realizing that it requires more than the excellent grades and MCAT scores. So, the book is not only about our success, but about our missteps and how we can help you and the new premeds in our circle avoid these missteps. This undertaking is not for the faint of heart. Medical school is one of the most difficult professional schools in which to gain admission, arguably, second only to Veterinary medical school. Vet school, we think, takes the prize as the most difficult to gain admission. It's not just that there are a lot less Veterinary medical schools available than allopathic medical schools; it's also that the requirements are a little stricter in some ways than medical school. Many students do not realize this. Some veterinary medical students have spent 6 application cycles trying to get into vet school. That is a lot of heartbreak! That is also a lot of determination that could have been directed elsewhere towards this goal.

If you intend on being part of the 1% then this book will serve as a blueprint for success. This book does not teach the application process. There are numerous resources for that when the time comes. This book will focus on the years leading up to the application during which time you are preparing academically and non-academically. This is for your high schooler, college freshman and sophomore who will be applying to medical school in their junior year of college. This book is for the gap year students, 'non-traditional' students and graduate students because the plan laid out here is still going to be the same. The only difference is that you have chosen a different time frame in which to apply and therefore will need to be current on the strategy.

Throughout the book we will be addressing parents as well as students. I think, while our students are altruistic in their endeavors to become a doctor (and this is good), they are naïve to the fact that this requires strategy. Parents understand the planning, strategy and opportunistic tactics that may be required to get to the head of the pack. Students do not have time for the strategy; they are much too busy studying. Try passing organic chemistry when you have four other science courses to deal with- it consumes you!

Starting from high school, everything your student does should be strategic. Start laying the groundwork early in high school. No, it is not too early because as soon as your student hits college, it is full throttle ahead, a non-stop path until they graduate medical school. It is a battle, and it requires strategy to turn you into a highly qualified candidate for medical school. But what is a 'highly qualified candidate'? Read on and let's get started.

As a pre-med student, I worked for 3 years in the chemistry lab with a great chem lab director. A few years later I found out she had gone to medical school. As a pre-med student, I also had a wonderful, extremely knowledgeable guidance counselor. A few years later I found out that she too had gone to medical school. Yes! The guidance counselor! They are both lovely women that were very encouraging and influential in my journey through college and into podiatric medical school, so I was happy and excited for them when I found out. But how interesting is it that they both were accepted into medical school? While I realize now that they may have always had the desire to be a physician, I also realized that they had figured out the formula. Yes, a formula for admission to medical school! At the same time, I also had a classmate named Jen. Jen was a 50-something year old mother of a medical doctor. I remember sitting next to her at our mock MCAT exam. We were giggling at something silly while waiting for the exam to start. Jen was accepted at a medical school in Mexico. Last I heard, she was back in the USA happily practicing. That was years ago of course. Jen knew the strategy because she had already employed it with her son who was a medical doctor. When the results of the strategy zigged, Jen zagged (to Mexico) and accomplished her goal of becoming a doctor.

There will be thousands of students with great GPA's and MCAT scores. Some of these students may even pay thousands of dollars to a coach or admissions consulting company to help them gain admission to medical school. However, they present to these experts with nothing else for them to work with. Then the student must play catch up to strengthen their resume. Whether you are a junior or a non-traditional student, you have worked hard to get to the point where you meet the academic requirements for medical school. To only have your goals derailed because you did not complete the non-academic requirements would be disappointing and costly! *Every application cycle that you delay is a year of physician income lost!*

Consider my student's friend Sue. Sue graduated college with a 3.8 science GPA and worked as a medical scribe for three years at a major urgent care center. Her goal was to become a Physician Assistant. We thought with her excellent academic standing and clinical work experience that she was the perfect applicant for physician assistant school or medical school. So, imagine our shock when she was denied acceptance to her first-choice school. She was later accepted into another great PA program in which she is happy. However, we had questions. Could it be that the school did not consider her experiences as well rounded or sufficient? Wasn't her strong academic credentials enough to overlook any other deficiencies in her application? We do not know what their reasoning was. We do know that we want to use time and strategy to prepare candidates so that there are no perceived gaps or holes in their applications. **The goal of this book is to make you so interesting a candidate that the medical school admissions committee will simply *want* to meet you!**

Here are some abbreviations used throughout the medical school application process that you should become familiar with now as a premed student.

ABBREVIATIONS TO KNOW

AACOMAS: American Association of Colleges of Osteopathic Medicine Application Service This is the centralized online application service for students applying to U.S. colleges of osteopathic medicine.

AACPM: The American Association of Colleges of Podiatric Medicine is a nationally recognized education organization that represents the nine accredited U.S. colleges of podiatric medicine

AACPMAS: The American Association of Colleges of Podiatric Medicine Application Service is the centralized application service for applicants to podiatric medical school.

AADSAS: The Associated American Dental School Application Service.

AAMC: The Association of American Medical Colleges is an organization of medical education
institutions. The AAMC administers the MCAT and runs AMCAS. www.aamc.org

AAPA: American Academy of Physician Assistants. www.aapa.org

AAVMC: Association of American Veterinary Medical Colleges

ADCOM: Admissions Committee, referring to the admissions committee of a medical school or a member of that committee

AMCAS: The American Medical College Application Service is

the online centralized
application for most medical schools in the US.

BCPM GPA: Biology, Chemistry, Physics, Mathematics GPA. This math/science GPA is
separated out as you apply to medical school.

CASPA: Centralized Application Service for Physician Assistants.

CASPer: Computer-based Assessment for Sampling Personal characteristics. It is a situational judgement test used by academic programs to help assess applicants for non-academic attributes or people skills like professionalism, communication, ethics, and empathy. Many medical schools are using this now. (Don't worry, it's not a test that you study for)

DAT: Dental School Admission Test. The DAT is required by all U.S. dental schools and measures academic ability, scientific understanding, and perceptual ability.

DO: Doctor of Osteopathic Medicine. Licensed physicians who practice in all areas of medicine, emphasizing a whole-person-approach to treatment and care that incorporates musculoskeletal manipulations.

FAP: The Fee Assistance Program provides access to the MCAT and the AMCAS for financially challenged students at reduced cost.
IMG: International Medical Graduates. These doctors have graduated from medical schools outside the USA and Canada. Also known as FMG

GRE: The Graduate Record Examinations is the test that students take to enter graduate school. Vet school and physician assistant school applicants also take this test.

MCAT: The Medical College Admission Test is a standardized, multiple-choice examination created to help medical school admissions offices assess your problem solving, critical thinking, and knowledge of natural, behavioral, and social science concepts and principles prerequisite to the study of medicine.

MSAR: The Medical School Admission Requirements is an online database that provides specific information, requirements, and statistics on medical schools in the United States and Canada that you can browse, search, sort and compare. You can use this to make an informed decision on which medical schools you would like to attend.

MSTP: Medical scientist training program. These programs lead to the combined MD/PhD degree

PS: Personal Statement. This is the essay that will be part of your medical school application.

SHPEP: Summer Health Professions Education Program. This program provides underrepresented students with experiences in the medical field. www.shpep.org

URM: Underrepresented in Medicine are those racial and ethnic populations underrepresented in the medical profession relative to their numbers in the general population.

MD: Doctor of Medicine is a physician who has had many years of training in the diagnosis,
treatment, and prevention of disease. An MD's training is in allopathic medicine.

TMDSAS: Texas Medical & Dental Schools Application Service is the online application for medical and dental schools in Texas. Texas does not subscribe to AMCAS.

VITA: Video interview tool. A new remote interview tool used by some medical schools where you create a video and the AAMC distributes to the schools. It is done in addition to the regular interview.

VMCAS: Veterinary Medical College Application Service. This is the centralized application service for applying to veterinary medical school.

VMSAR: Veterinary Medical School Admissions Requirements is an online database that provides specific information, requirements, and statistics on veterinary medical schools in the United States and Internationally that you can browse, search, sort and compare. You can use this to make an informed decision on which Veterinary medical schools you would like to attend.

CHAPTER 1 **WHAT DO MEDICAL SCHOOLS REALLY WANT TO SEE IN A CANDIDATE?**

So, what are medical schools looking for in a candidate? We know that they want to see that you have good grades and a strong MCAT score and these two may be the most important screening factors. There are occasions where a candidate may have a not-so-great GPA or MCAT score and they are still granted admission to medical school. Why? It is because the ADCOMS see value in these candidates' other attributes. What are these other attributes that they are seeking to find as they comb through your application?

When asked what they look for in a student, many of the schools will say something like this: "We take a holistic approach in evaluating applications, emphasizing medical, humanitarian, research, employment, leadership and other diverse life experiences. Most successful applicants also have cumulative and science GPAs around 'abc' and an MCAT score of at least 'xyz'." Or- "We do a holistic review and look beyond GPA and MCAT scores". What is a *Holistic* Review? In an AAMC interview, one student admissions committee member says this about her training as an interviewer: "Our training also included applying holistic review, which means looking beyond candidates' GPA and MCAT® scores to their attributes and experiences, like intellectual curiosity, maturity, and community service. We were encouraged to pair holistic review with a focus on our school's mission to create a diverse class with members who will help improve health in the communities and regions the school serves." (You can read the rest of the interview here: https://www.aamc.org/news-insights/insights/what-its-be-student-admissions-committee)

These other attributes that the schools look for are specifically laid out in the AAMC's 15 core competencies. According to the AAMC, a competency is defined as an observable behavior that combines knowledge, skills, values, and attitudes related to a specific activity. The Competencies for Entering Medical Students include 15 competencies in four categories:

1) Interpersonal competencies are service orientation, social skills, cultural competence, teamwork, and oral communication; 2) Intrapersonal competencies are ethical responsibility to self and others, reliability and dependability, resiliency and adaptability, and capacity for improvement; 3) Thinking and reasoning competencies are critical thinking, quantitative reasoning, scientific inquiry, and written communication; and 4) Science competencies are living systems and human behavior.

Here is a list of the 15 competencies listed in their 4 categories:

Interpersonal Competencies-

Service Orientation: Demonstrates a desire to help others and sensitivity to others' needs and feelings; demonstrates a desire to alleviate others' distress; recognizes and acts on his/her responsibilities to society; locally, nationally, and globally.

Social Skills: Demonstrates an awareness of others' needs, goals, feelings, and the ways that social and behavioral cues affect peoples' interactions and behaviors; adjusts behaviors appropriately in response to these cues; treats others with respect.

Cultural Competence: Demonstrates knowledge of socio-cultural factors that affect interactions and behaviors; shows an appreciation and respect for multiple dimensions of diversity; recognizes and acts on the obligation to inform one's own judgment; engages diverse and competing perspectives as a resource for learning, citizenship, and work; recognizes and appropriately addresses bias in themselves and others; interacts effectively with people from diverse backgrounds.

Teamwork: Works collaboratively with others to achieve shared goals; shares information and knowledge with others and provides feedback; puts team goals ahead of individual goals.

Oral Communication: Effectively conveys information to others using spoken words and sentences; listens effectively; recognizes potential communication barriers and adjusts approach or clarifies information as needed.

Intrapersonal Competencies

Ethical Responsibility to Self and Others: Behaves in an honest and ethical manner; cultivates personal and academic integrity; adheres to ethical principles and follows rules and procedures; resists peer pressure to engage in unethical behavior and encourages others to behave in honest and ethical ways; develops and demonstrates ethical and moral reasoning.

Reliability and Dependability: Consistently fulfills obligations in a timely and satisfactory manner; takes responsibility for personal actions and performance.

Resilience and Adaptability: Demonstrates tolerance of stressful or changing environments or situations and adapts effectively to them; is persistent, even under difficult situations; recovers from setbacks.

Capacity for Improvement: Sets goals for continuous improvement and for learning new concepts and skills; engages in reflective practice for improvement; solicits and responds appropriately to feedback.

Thinking and Reasoning Competencies

Critical Thinking: Uses logic and reasoning to identify the strengths and weaknesses of alternative solutions, conclusions, or approaches to problems.

Quantitative Reasoning: Applies quantitative reasoning and appropriate mathematics to describe or explain phenomena in the natural world.

Scientific Inquiry: Applies knowledge of the scientific process to integrate and synthesize information, solve problems and formulate research questions and hypotheses; is facile in the language of the sciences and uses it to participate in the discourse of science and explain how scientific knowledge is discovered and validated.

Written Communication: Effectively conveys information to others using written words and sentences.

Science Competencies

Living Systems: Applies knowledge and skill in the natural sciences to solve problems related to molecular and macro systems including biomolecules, molecules, cells, and organs.

Human Behavior: Applies knowledge of the self, others, and social systems to solve problems related to the psychological, socio-cultural, and biological factors that influence health and well-being.

Start inculcating these qualities in your students now. These qualities develop and show up in academics, research, publications, volunteerism, community service, clinical experiences and MCAT scores. They are then reflected in the way these are presented and highlighted in your medical school application, letters of recommendation, personal statement, essays and interviews.

CHAPTER 2 HIGH SCHOOL - IS IT TOO EARLY   TO GET STARTED?

How to get into medical school from high school

High school is a great time for students to grow their passion for medicine and to start planning their career journey. As you will see later, this can actually be the time that your student secures an acceptance into medical school! So, it is not too early to get started. Achieving good grades and SAT/ACT scores along with participating in extra-curricular activities are important for personal development and for admission to college. As a premed student, however, you should include some clinical or scientific activities. These activities can cement your decision to pursue medicine or reveal, early on, that medicine is not for you. These activities will later demonstrate to medical school admissions committees that you had an early, avid interest in medicine. This early interest is not required for medical school acceptance (some successful applicants decide on medicine much later in their lives) but it can be an interesting and impressive aspect of *your* application. Here is a short list of some activities that can give you medical/clinical exposure and scientific experiences while in high school:

Physician Shadowing – This involves following a doctor around as they go about their daily workday activities: seeing and examining patients and if you are lucky you can observe procedures. Shadowing a doctor can help you to decide if you are truly interested in medicine and interested in providing hands on patient care to sick people. Many students at this stage discover that they cannot stand the site of blood or open wounds and realize that this may not actually be their life's passion. Better to discover this early than later! But realistically, at this stage, expect any hands-on exposure to be limited or nonexistent due to liability.

Volunteer Work- Any of your local hospitals should have a volunteer program to which your student can apply. It would be great to start this in Junior year of High School or at least after your student turns 16 years old. Some states may require a work permit for students under 18 years old. Vaccination records showing up to date vaccines and a negative PPD test (test for tuberculosis) will be required before you start work. Your student should be able to pick their schedule according to hospital available shifts. If you are an aspiring future veterinarian, volunteer work is a must at this stage. Many vet schools require 200 hours of small and large animal experience, so get to work from now so that you are not pressured towards the end.

I know students may want to do volunteer work in other fields, and they should, but remember our battle strategy. This is one of the strategic moves that shows early interest in the medical field and true empathy for patients.

Summer Programs – Along with your guidance counselors and science teachers, the AAMC is a great resource to find a medicine related summer program. Here is the link to search their database for a suitable program: https://services.aamc.org/summerprograms/ Select High School level.

Here we have listed a few of our favorite programs:

Cornell University Summer College – 'The Cornell University Research Apprenticeship in the Biological Sciences **(RABS)** offers a small number of serious, research-oriented students the rare opportunity to join a top-notch laboratory at one of the world's leading research institutions.' This program is for junior and senior high school students interested in biological research. 'During this innovative, intensive, and highly selective program, you'll become part of the renowned biomedical research community at Cornell's Ithaca campus, studying under the guidance of distinguished Cornell faculty members as you pursue research in an area of your choosing. Students will develop their research skills, becoming familiar with the lab procedures, protocols, techniques, and equipment used in cutting-edge facilities. Also, they will attend seminars on topics such as biology, medicine, and science ethics. All the while, they work closely with some of Cornell's leading professors, postdoctoral fellows, and graduate and undergraduate researchers. Here is the link https://sce.cornell.edu/precollege/summer-college

The program is highly prestigious and upon completion the student earns 6 college credits and a Cornell university transcript. As you can imagine, the program is costly. As you can also imagine, acceptance into this program would be a game changer.

MITES Program at MIT- Minority Introduction to Engineering and Science (MITES) oeop.mit.edu is an intensive six-week residential academic enrichment program for about 80 promising high school juniors who intend to pursue careers in science, engineering, and entrepreneurship, especially those from minority backgrounds and other underrepresented segments of the population. The program is free of charge to participating students, not including transportation.

STEP-UP NIH - STEP-UP is a great program offered by the National Institutes of Health (NIH) specifically the National Institute of Diabetes and Digestive and Kidney Diseases (The NIDDK). The program is an 8 to 10 week full-time paid research experience. The goal of the program is for students from underrepresented backgrounds to be exposed to and participate in biomedical, behavioral, clinical and social science research. Your student gets to choose an approved institution or mentor in their hometown or within commuting distance. If you cannot find a researcher on your own, the program will match you with one. My student was able to work with a wonderful Pediatrician who did biomedical research at Albert Einstein School of Medicine in Bronx, New York. This doctor also worked at Montefiore Hospital, so she made sure she was also exposed to a clinical experience. At the end of the program the students can present their work PowerPoint presentation at the research symposium at the NIH in Bethesda, Maryland. Also, in my student's year, their work was published in a medical journal. As you can imagine, this program provides a powerful experience to a young premed student. The application deadline is usually in early February for high school students and college students. The application includes a compelling essay and three letters of recommendation. The essay should convey an interest in medical research   Does your student have an interest in research? Apply! Does your student have absolutely no interest in research? Apply! This is a battle, remember? Well, this is part of the strategy.

HiSTEP is also an NIH program for high schoolers. www.training.nih.gov/histep

Whitehead Institute for Biomedical Research Spring Lecture Series – Now this program I absolutely loved! Whitehead Institute is a Harvard-MIT affiliated institution that offers a 3-day program to High school Sophomores and Juniors during spring break. There is no fee or tuition. These are 3 days packed with an unparalleled world-class experience in the arena of scientific research. The spaces are limited, so getting your student into this program requires some strategy in of itself. The link to apply is usually released sometime after midnight on the pre- announced date. Before this date, try to get a hold of the short 1- page application/recommendation that is required for a teacher and parent to sign off on. Get it completed. Then, on midnight of the open application date, you have to stalk the website and wait for the link to go active. Yes, I've done this- stayed up until 2-3am on 3 different times with success! Once it does go live, follow all instructions to upload or fax over your application immediately and your student should get in. The reason for the madness is that, as I mentioned before, space is limited. Acceptance is on a first come- first served basis. So, this was my strategy for getting my two students into this world-renowned institution. They were introduced to and exposed to scientific research, participated in labs including dissections and running PCRs. Here is the link for this program: https://wi.mit.edu/program/spring-lecture-series-high-school-students

Whitehead has other programs so please explore their website. www.wi.mit.edu

Note that some programs require an essay showing your interest and passion for science or medicine. It may be a good idea to do your hospital volunteer work and a physician shadowing before you apply. A science fair project or community-based project are great also. This way you can *show* your interest and not just *say* that you are interested. Other programs want to encourage students into STEM or medicine careers and no prior interest is necessary.

AP Advanced Placement courses - Do as many AP courses as you can whether it is in the science field or not. Here's why: If you take an AP course in a non- science subject such as English Literature for example and score at least a 3 on the placement exam, it will count as college credits towards English 101, e.g. So, now, you do not have to waste precious time taking it as a college freshman! And time is so precious if you are a premed student.

If you take a science AP course and score at least a 3 on the exam, it will count as college credits towards a level 1 science course. Now that is a major win, weight off the shoulder and room to breathe for a premed student. However, you better have gotten a good grade because it will appear on your transcript when you apply to medical school!

Some other points to note:

An AP science course sometimes may not be at the same level as the equivalent college course, so you may find the level 2 course to be difficult. How to tell? Go over the college's course syllabus and compare and see if the material was covered in detail in your AP course.

Any AP course that your college accepts will save you money on paying for college credits. Please note that some schools require a score of 4 on The AP exams. Also, some schools may not accept certain AP subjects as college credit. Make sure to consider these factors when you choose your colleges.

BS/MD programs

This is one of the reasons we say high school is not too early to start planning – The Bachelor of Science/Arts combined with the Doctor of Medicine program. These programs accept a student into their college with a guaranteed spot in the school's associated or affiliated medical school. There is no application or admissions process later on, as the student is already accepted into medical school. Imagine being guaranteed a seat in medical school right out of high school! Not so fast- the guaranteed acceptance to medical school is contingent upon maintaining a certain GPA and for some schools- MCAT scores. These programs also require that you participate in other medical career enhancing activities. Some BS/MD programs are the full 8 years (4 years of college and 4 years of medical school) while others are condensed into 6 or 7 years. A few programs are 9 years. You are also committed to this particular school throughout your undergraduate and medical school journey.

This is a program designed for high achieving, highly focused and motivated high school students who know definitively that they want to become a medical doctor- in other words, you. A typical candidate would have shown excellent academic performance with a great GPA and SAT/ACT scores. They would have shown an early passion and motivation for medicine via hospital or other clinical volunteer work, scientific or medical research experience via summer programs and other programs as discussed in the previous sections and upcoming chapters. They would also have shown an interest in community work.

Students apply to the BS/MD program in high school in their junior year, just as they would apply to college. However, there will be an interview for these programs. Students should be prepared to answer the same "Why medicine?" question that college seniors must answer on their medical school personal statements and interviews. College seniors obviously would have a few more years of experience with which to tackle this most important question. The BS/MD candidate must ramp up and match their experiences with their early choice of a medical career to be able to answer this all-important question.

BS/MD programs are few and highly competitive with each offering only a few spots each year. Their requirements vary. You must research these schools carefully to choose a program that is right for you. There are many articles but just a few resources available for you to do this. You could try directly contacting a school in which you are interested to see if they have a BS/MD program. See the AAMC's **list of programs** at the end of the book.

Also, we love this article by PrepScholar: https://blog.prepscholar.com/ba-md-bs-md-programs-list

If you are a high school student interested in the BS/MD program you can benefit from purchasing the MSAR database from the AAMC as it lists the current year's BS/MD programs and their requirements.

CHAPTER 3   COLLEGE - WHAT SHOULD YOU BE DOING?

If your student is already in college and missed out on the high school strategies, no worries. There are still plenty opportunities to build on strategy. Also, you now qualify for more opportunities and can appreciate and grow from them. In this chapter we will list the activities that the AAMC has recommended for premed students. While in college you want to start working on building those 15 core competencies we mentioned earlier. Besides the learning experience, the student should start to pay attention to how each clinical or non-clinical experience challenges them, helps them to grow and how the activity has changed them. As you do each extra- curricular activity related to medicine, ask yourself 'is this for me?', 'am I enjoying this?'. The answers to these questions will cement your interest and dedication to medicine or will let you know that some or all aspects of medicine are just not for you. The goal is not just to impress admissions committees but to impress yourself! This self-questioning will help you form the answer to the most important question that all medical schools want to know about you- Why Medicine?

Gaining clinical experience, doing volunteer work and community service show that you are a serious candidate who understands the field of medicine and health care. It shows that you care about people and about your community. It shows that you understand healthcare disparities in vulnerable populations, an understanding that will be reflected in the quality of care that you, later, will provide to *all* your patients. Medical schools want to know this about you before they invest four years in you.

Premed and Prehealth Advisors

Throughout you academic and application journey work with

your premed or prehealth advisor. They have a wealth of information and experience from which you will benefit. They will help to keep you on track with your course requirements. They should be your first source to find your activities and programs. Meet with them at the beginning and end of each semester. We have heard the disappointing stories about advisors who are not encouraging or even dissuade students from applying to medical school. Unfortunately, we have experienced such advisors in this family, were quickly able to identify them and neutralize them. Goodbye. There are *many* great advisors out there who can guide you straight into medical school. I see many of these advisors at medical school fairs trying to learn the latest information and advocating heavily on behalf of their students. If you cannot find someone like this to work with you once you have announced your intentions to apply to medical school, you can contact the NAAHP to find an advisor. The National Association of Advisors for the Health Professions is an organization of health professions advisors at colleges and universities throughout the United States, and abroad. They offer free counseling services to students who cannot access them at their schools. You can request an advisor at www.naahp.org

Volunteer Work

The **volunteer work** started in high school should be continued. This time the goal is different. You should be trying to get exposure to clinical care of the patient. Prepping patients, assisting patients, comforting and talking to patients- these are all aspects of clinical care. Again, try the local hospital or maybe a clinic near or on campus depending on where your college is located. You could also volunteer to assist at blood drives, health screenings and health fairs.

Join **the Medical Reserve Corp** in your city as a non-medical or medical volunteer. Their focus is on public health, community health initiatives, emergencies and disaster preparedness. You will do a short training to get on board. You can then volunteer for their different activities and training exercises. It is another way to demonstrate community activism and leadership in a medical setting. Visit https://mrc.hhs.gov/

PHYSICIAN SHADOWING

As mentioned before, physician shadowing involves observing a physician as she works throughout the day to get an idea of what is involved in a doctor's workday. If you have already done shadowing in high school please do not spend too much time shadowing a doctor now unless you really feel there is a further benefit to you. It does not count as clinical experience hours and you should be aiming for that closer interaction with patients at this point. If you choose to continue shadowing, try establishing a relationship this time with the doctor and staff. You will value this relationship later as a source for advice and letters of recommendation.

Jobs

To be honest, any job that you enjoy doing or need to do because it pays the bills is going to be fine. It's not so much what job you do that's important, it's what experiences you can take away from that job. As one medical school admissions officer pointed out, physicians are not always the leaders on a team! You need to show that you can work with a team, take instructions, follow orders. That job at McDonalds or that waitress job can cultivate these skills and you should include these job experiences in your medical school applications. However, there are some jobs that you can do that will help you to also accomplish or fulfill some of your *required* extracurricular activities like being a medical scribe or a lab assistant. I worked in the chemistry lab most of the four years I was in college, ironically so did my daughter. College work study is financial aid that places you in a job, usually on campus and in your field of study. This is a great way to get placed in a job in the field of science. Here are some other **jobs** that will give you great **scientific** or **clinical** exposure and experience:

EMT – Emergency Medical Technician (basic, volunteer)

CNA – Certified Nursing Assistant

Medical Scribe - virtual or onsite

Lab assistant – bio lab or chem lab on campus

Research assistant – on campus or at another institution

Clinical Research Assistant – Train to be a CRA. Visit @clin.trial.talk for everything CRA

Lab technician – Hospital or diagnostic lab. Visit @medicine-mons for her lab tech/premed experience

LEADERSHIP

One of the skills that admissions committees would like to see a candidate possess is leadership skills. As a student doctor, resident or attending doctor you will often be leading a team. It may be a team of college students, medical students following the resident, or an attending in charge of a patient care team or in the operating room. These groups are looking to you for knowledge, discernment, planning and delegation.

One way to demonstrate this skill is by participating in a club on campus and holding an active position in the club. For example, you can be president, treasurer etc. of the pre-med or pre-vet club.

Get involved with your campus' Healthy Campus Initiative (HCI) or help start a Healthy Campus Initiative at your college.

Another activity is community health awareness initiatives. What health issues are there in your community that are of concern to you? Are there health care disparities in your community? Create an awareness campaign and present a poster about it.

Leadership can also be demonstrated in smaller ways during your everyday activities. Directing class projects, organizing study groups or trips to premed conferences all require good leadership and organizational skills. Be prepared to relate these stories when answering interview questions on leadership. It's easy to forget the smaller, equally as meaningful activities that you did.

Some schools may want to see that you have a certain number of hours of clinical experience or volunteer work, other schools do not. You can always check by calling, visiting their website or checking the MSAR to see what the school's policy is. What all medical schools *do* value is that you have been consistent in these activities throughout your premed journey. So, don't rush to do everything at once, but do start early so that you can do what is interesting and fulfilling to you. You will be happier and even find yourself contributing and making a positive change in whatever activity you participate.

AAMC

Put aside time and spend a few days going through the AAMC website. It is gold! Don't forget to revisit it each year. The AAMC administers the MCAT and runs AMCAS, the centralized application service for medical schools. AMCAS is like the medical school version of the Common App used for college applications. Applicants input all their coursework, test scores, research projects, awards, and extracurricular activities. They also upload the personal statement. AMCAS then formats all the information, creating an application and transmits it to all the medical schools that you have selected.

The AAMC also puts out the Medical School Admission Requirements (MSAR) each year. It is an online database where you can browse, search, sort and compare current information about medical schools. It is one of the tools that will help you to maximize your chances for admission and choose schools where you will be happy and can achieve your goals maximize your chances for admission.

PREMEDICAL CONFERENCES AND FAIRS

Attending these is a must. Premedical conferences or medical school fairs are events occurring throughout the year and attending them is extremely valuable. They bring together dozens of medical schools, veterinary medical schools and osteopathic medical schools, along with their admissions representatives and their medical students all under one roof. These events present the opportunity for pre-med students to visit the booth of a school, ask questions and gather information from admission reps and students who may be on the admissions committees. This is gold, especially if the student can create a rapport with the school's reps by following up with a thank you email and follow up questions or asking for new advice. However, the goal is to gather as much information as possible while you are there. I love talking to the students who are on the admissions committee because their advice and tips is more forthcoming and brutally honest as they are less constrained than an administrative rep. Most of the fairs are free while some require a small fee to attend. The AAMC has a free virtual fair once a year that is great for those who are unable to travel to fairs or individual schools. There are workshops and panel discussions on a variety of topics such as MCAT preparation, financing your application and medical career, the application process and resources for applicants. This format also has the advantage in that you can see the questions from other students and the answers from the reps. Attend these conferences, get the advice, enjoy the freebies but most of all-follow up new contacts with thank you emails. At a virtual fair a few months ago, I saw one young man mention to the admissions rep of a school that he heard there were a few more interviews this season at the school. It was the end of the application cycle and he was worried because he had not received an interview yet. This was his dream school. He then asked whether he still had a chance of being selected for an interview. The admissions rep replied yes, they were still interviewing to fill a few seats. I really hope that he used his real name! (your name and optional photo appear when you ask a question). What are the chances that the rep may remember his name later when selecting interviewees? What if he followed up with a simple thank you email? I wish I could be a fly on the wall for that one. I did not know him, but I was proud of that bold move. Follow-up with thank you emails and perhaps a follow-up question for contacts that you make. You never know who is watching or who may remember you. Strategy!

CHAPTER 4 RESEARCH - THE HOLY GRAIL

At the recent Columbia University Medical School Fair in New York City, we had the opportunity to speak with admissions officers and representatives from several schools (we will talk more on medical school fairs later). One of the topics on our minds was whether scientific or clinical research experience is *the holy grail* in med school acceptance. Some schools want to see that the candidate has research experience. Most agreed that scientific research experience was not a requirement for admission to medical school unless you were applying to an MD/PhD program. However, they did say that about 75% of admitted students had done some research. One admin said that the trend may be student driven! Either way, we are not gambling here. Research is part of our strategy for gaining admission to medical school. Make it enjoyable. Do something that interests you. All research does not have to be scientific but let it be something that contributes to a community's social well-being and health. Let's get started.

One of the best ways to get involved in scientific research is to ask a professor who has a lab. See which professor's research genuinely interests you and approach them. Also, some schools may participate in government research initiatives like the Minority Biomedical Research Support Program or Maximizing Access to Research Careers Ask your premed advisor. If you are unable to secure a research position in your school or would prefer to explore outside opportunities, there are scores of research opportunities across the country. Here are a couple of programs that we recommend:
The National Science Foundation has numerous research opportunities in institutions around the country. Check with

your school first to see if they participate. Also use this link to see other research programs with the NSF www.nsf.gov

STEM Undergrads website is a source that lists federally funded STEM research opportunities for undergraduate students. https://stemundergrads.science.gov/

NIH STEP-UP Again, this is a great program offered by the National Institute of Health (NIH) specifically the National Institute of Diabetes and Digestive and Kidney Diseases (The NIDDK). For the undergraduate, premed student, the program is an 8 -10 week full-time paid research experience. The goal of the program is for students from underrepresented backgrounds to be exposed to and participate in biomedical, behavioral, clinical and social science research. Your student gets to choose an approved institution or mentor in their hometown or within commuting distance. If you cannot find a researcher on your own, the program will match you with one. At the end of the program the student will present their work in a Power-Point presentation at the National Institutes of Health (NIH) in Maryland. As mentioned before there may be an opportunity to have your mentor's work published in a medical journal. The deadline for undergrads is usually early February. https://www.niddk.nih.gov/research-funding/research-programs/

NIDDK research programs- These are open to all students from all backgrounds www.niddk.nih.gov click on research and funding.

NIH other programs- www.training.nih.gov/programs/ugsp/scholarshipbenefits

NASA has great research internships for STEM majors also, starting at the high school level.
https://intern.nasa.gov/

Summer Programs- Summer Health Professions Education Program, the SHPEP program is another great program for underrepresented students who are in their freshman and sophomore year of college. 'The FREE six-week summer enrichment program helps college students enhance their academic proficiency and career development opportunities in a health profession. Participation in the summer enrichment program may better position students for acceptance into advanced-degree programs.'   'All student housing costs, meals, and travel to and from the program site are covered by the program. Students are awarded a $600 stipend (raised to $1000 this year due to virtual program) for successfully completing the program.' We love a program that pays the student! The nice thing about the SHPEP program is that it is offered in 12 different institutions around the country. So, students around the country can participate in this opportunity. One official said that 65% of SHPEP students go on to be accepted into medical school. For further information visit www.shpep.org Also the deadline is early February.

See the addendum for a list of research programs across the country.

If your PI is ready and in agreement to **publish your work**, here are some student- friendly journals in which student can have their work published (recommended by the Institute for Health Care Improvement):

The American Medical Student Research Journal was created by medical students to give future physician-scientists the opportunity to develop the critical thinking skills needed to succeed in academia and clinical practice. (The) journal is authored, reviewed, and edited by medical students working under the guidance of faculty mentors. http://amsrj.org/index.php?journal=amsrj&page=index

Einstein Journal of Biology and Medicine (EJBM)
http://www.einstein.yu.edu/publications/einstein-journal-biology-medicine/
The Harvard Medical Student Review
http://www.hmsreview.org/?page_id=19

Harvard Public Health Review
http://harvardpublichealthreview.org/

International Journal of Medical Students
http://www.ijms.info/ojs/index.php/IJMS/about/submissions#.VADFAfldV1A

Student BMJ
http://student.bmj.com/student/static-pages.html?pageId=2

*** See the research section in the Covid Pivot Chapter

The American Association of Medical Colleges notes 'that with ever-increasing globalization in medicine there is growing interest on the part of medical students and medical schools to integrate international electives into their medical education. Global experiences enable students to interact with different patient populations, develop cross-cultural understanding, and learn about health systems in other nations.' Well, how impressive would it be to start gaining this experience as a pre-medical student? Studying or volunteering abroad offers unique opportunities to learn in your specific field of study and to grow through these amazing experiences. Participating in one of these programs can be an admissions game-changer for an applicant to medical school. The advantage with these programs is that the student gets to do more hands-on work than they can do here at home. For example, a pre-veterinarian student may get to assist in animal neutering, spading and other surgical procedures. As part of one program, premed students can observe cases in the operating room. This would not be allowed in most practices or hospitals here in the US due to medical-legal limitations.

The disadvantage may be the cost involved. However, many programs have scholarships or tuition payment plans available. There are numerous travel-abroad programs starting from the high school level. Here we will discuss a few programs that we like.

Join Atlantis is a program that allows premed students to shadow doctors in 20 hours per week in Europe or Latin America. The programs run between 1.5 to 8 weeks during the winter and summer breaks. Scholarships are available. The students rotate through different specialties to gain exposure to various medical practices and procedures. Some specialties include internal medicine, emergency medicine, oncology and pediatrics.

Volunteering Solutions provides great and affordable projects in 11 countries including the Philippines, Thailand, Cambodia, Vietnam, Tanzania, South Africa, Ghana, Uganda, Kenya, Peru and Costa Rica. 'Travel and be a part of a pre-med volunteering project in 2020 and gain international work experience that will immensely benefit your career as well as give you an opportunity to serve the underprivileged societies in these developing countries'.

FIMRC is a non- profit organization that works to improve health care access in developing nations by providing clinical care, community outreach and health education. Along with health care professionals and other partnerships, this is accomplished with the help of volunteers who travel around the world. Volunteers start at the high school level and up. Visit www.firmc.org for more information.

The pre-med students who join as volunteers are usually placed at hospitals and clinics in rural or suburban areas where there is inadequate staff. You will mostly work under the supervision of doctors, nurses as well as support staff and assist them in the treatment of patients. Being a part of any of these projects will also teach you more about the healthcare scenario and how economically disadvantaged populations still face challenges to get access to quality healthcare in developing countries. Visit www.firmc.org for more information.

Loop Abroad is a wonderful program for pre-veterinary students, ranging from the high school level to college. Loop Abroad provides hands on veterinary courses and volunteer jobs with pre-vets in mind. Students receive large and small animal experience, working with the endangered elephant populations, dogs, cats and a variety of wildlife. Students can work in clinics where they learn and practice new clinical skills. Locations include Thailand, South Africa, Australia,

Central America and South America. Loop Abroad offers 14-week semester abroad programs and 6-week volunteer abroad programs. College credits and some scholarships are available. Next to biological research, I think Loop Abroad played a big part in my student's acceptance to vet school. https://www.loopabroad.com/

Note, when you volunteer abroad go with the mindset that it is a privilege and honor to be in another country, experiencing its culture. Yes, you are a volunteer, not a tourist, but you will be more or less learning rather than helping at this point. They can certainly survive without you! Learn as much as you can about the culture, their approach to healthcare, and how they deliver healthcare to patients.

Finally, here are the words of one student who had a great perspective on her volunteer abroad program:
"Remember, there will be thousands of students with the same GPA, MCAT or GRE scores as you. Those are important numbers that adcoms use to *screen out* candidates; your extra-curricular experiences are what make you *stand out*."

CHAPTER 6 **PASSION PROJECTS - LIGHT THE FUSE!**

Are we boring you? Then maybe we can light a fuse and blow it up several notches for you with a ***passion project***!

Have you ever been told to follow your passion? Since you're planning on applying to med school, you've almost got it covered! But let's not forget about your other interests. They're just as important to your journey. In fact, showing admissions how dedicated you are to your passions will not only make you a well-rounded candidate but the ideal medical school student. When applying to med school you're always looking for ways to stay ahead of the game and stand out from the competition. Admissions look for applications that have extra-curricular activities, volunteer hours, and research experience, but they are also trying to find out what makes you tick, your passions and your values. However, there are only so many places to volunteer and clubs to join during high school and college. Also, much of your activities are learning and growing experiences and often leave little chance to make a direct impact in people's lives. One of the important aspects of clinical and non-clinical activities is how *you* have impacted other people. Passion projects gives you the freedom to do that.

A consistent long-term project shows ADCOMS who you are, and it packs a powerful punch! A passion project is ongoing work, research and activity about a particular hobby, topic or cause a student has chosen to pursue. This is a project that you brainstorm, create, start and finish. It should be aligned with your strengths and genius, with your personal values. It should be something that perhaps you already do or think about doing in your free time that excites you, something that you would do for free. This is a way to showcase your character and personality through a project with purpose of your own design. As a future doctor, this is an excellent way to display your dedication, responsibility, creativity, and leadership—traits that you need in the real world and in the medical field. Your passion of choice adds value to you as a person.

Admissions committee will see the application of someone who is ready and willing to save lives and someone who is capable of making a difference in the world. The project reflects your ability to create your own opportunities and take initiative. In med school, everyone brings something to the table. When educating the next generation of doctors, schools don't want to accept the exact same type of student, they want a diverse group of people who can learn from and teach one another. Each candidate should be able to add value to their class that no other student can.

Choose to dedicate time on your med school journey to pursue something that you are strongly passionate about. Passion projects are designed to express your commitment to something you truly care about in the world. Does anything come to mind? Do you advocate for building more homeless shelters in your local town? Does your grandparent have Alzheimer's and you've decided to interview the family members of other patients who have the same disease, or form a support group? Have you been following the rise of cryptocurrency and know more than your parents do about the future of economics? Are you great at gaining followers and subscribers on YouTube or Instagram and hold the most valuable secrets to social media marketing? Is mental health among students something that concerns you? Are you constantly in the lab working on your research? Approach your professor about publishing! Do you play the bass guitar and want to share your passion by giving lessons? See how easy brainstorming can be for ideas and how simple it can be to apply your interests into actions?

You can take action immediately on any of these topics. Creating a website, Instagram, twitter, YouTube, Facebook, blog,

club, business, writing an ebook, or forming a nonprofit organization, and more can be done to kick off your project. Learn
to delegate and outsource some of the work along the way. The
more original and impressive your ideas are, the more irresist-
ible you will be to admissions. Unlike your other activities
your passion project will be mentioned throughout your entire
application, kind of like a theme. This will allow admissions
committee members to get a sense of who you are and how
much this project meant to you. Think about how interesting your interview will be knowing you've spent a significant
amount of time doing your own independent project that you
can't wait to talk about. The success of organizing your own
passion project will leave you feeling proud, accomplished, and
confident—perfectly equipped for your role as a medical student.

Remember as kids you would have dreams of growing up to be a ballerina and a doctor at the same time or a fireman/baseball player or an astronaut/sanitation worker? The well-meaning adults would tell you that it could not be done, that you had to pick just one career. Well, they were right and wrong. As a pre-med student you have the freedom to pursue any college major of interest to you. Medical schools report that their admitted students come from a wide variety of academic backgrounds-dance, music, engineering, language arts and more. Medical schools say that these students bring unique insight and perspective to the field of medicine. While a student who majors in the sciences may indicate a long-term commitment to the field of science and medicine, a student who pursues their interest or passion is equally impressive.

So, what do these students from different academic backgrounds all have in common that got them accepted into medical school? They had all completed the required pre-requisite science and mathematics courses that all medical schools require. More importantly, they all did extremely well in these courses or at least showed a pattern of improving grades as they progressed.

Required Premed Courses – Here we will list the courses that most schools require. These courses must be completed by the time you apply to medical school. There are some exceptions depending on the school. Always research the academic requirements for the schools to which you are applying. The **MSAR** will help you with this and will be discussed later. You do not want to be scrambling to complete a course at the last minute. As fate would have it, the course most likely will not be available! And you are not leaving this battle up to fate, are you?

Also, make sure you have taken the courses that will be on the MCAT exam by the time you are ready to take the exam. Work with your guidance counselor to make sure you are registered for the correct courses at the correct time to meet your goals.

Some medical schools do not like to see that you took a science course or other major non-science prerequisite in the summer or winter break. Admission committees want to see that you can handle a full schedule of courses during the fall and spring semesters. It reflects how well you can handle the medical school curriculum. (If you have already taken a couple of science courses over the summer it is not a total deal breaker. Keep moving forward!)

Medical School Prerequisite Courses

- Biology 1 & 2 with lab
- General chemistry 1 & 2 with lab
- Physics 1 & 2
- Organic chemistry 1 & 2
- Biochemistry
- Genetics
- Calculus 1 & 2
- Psychology
- English
- Microbiology (some medical and vet schools)
- Animal Nutrition (some vet schools)
- Animal Science (some vet schools)

Maintaining a high GPA

Not every premed student will do well in the beginning obviously. All is not lost, however. As we mentioned before, a struggling student must demonstrate an upward trend in their grades. If you got a 'B' in Biology 101, try for an 'A' in Biology 102. If you got a 'C' in Organic Chemistry 1 try for a 'B' in Organic Chemistry 2. It shows a commitment to excelling and gaining a better grasp of the subject matter. These are some of the cognitive skills that ADCOMs want to see in you since they are predictors of how well you will perform *academically* in medical school. Medical schools cannot afford to have students drop out in the first or second year. It has a negative effect on their finances and status. They will want to make sure that you have what it takes, academically, to get through the rigorous medical school curriculum. **GPA and MCAT scores- these are the numbers that will get you through the door.** So how do you maintain a high grade point average? This will be mainly up to you, but we have a few strategies:

Discover your style of learning and capitalize on it (Metacognition). Too many students suffer needlessly and perform poorly simply because their style of learning has not been identified by them or by teachers in the early years. The main learning styles are identified as auditory, visual, kinesthetic, reading/writing and combinations of these. There is controversy about learning styles and their use though. However, we know that we learn subject matter in different ways. The way you learn math may be different from the way you learn and retain biology subject matter. Pay attention to how you learn and retain for each subject. Identify these differences so that you can adjust your study habits to maximize your most efficient (not enjoyable) learning abilities. Therefore, don't just sit there, *only* writing notes for *every* course. Apply **the 80/20 rule** and **Learn key concepts**. This rule, also known as the Pareto Rule, says that just 20% of your activities will produce 80% of your results. Simon Lee of Life-Hack says this applies to learning also- if we can identify the key concept (the 20%) behind what we are learning, this will the unlock everything to understanding that subject matter (the 80%). Of course, this will not apply to everything we learn in our premed courses, but it can be applied to every subject and you will know when to use it.

Do **mnemonics** work for you? **Encoding specificity**, where you learn something around one context and later retrieve the memory by the same context cue?

Spaced repetition and **active recall** work well for many students and is incorporated into some learning tools. Also, when you do take notes, handwrite them as opposed to typing them, or at least use an app like Notability, and an Apple pencil, you will retain better this way.

Lastly, take advantage of your recorded lectures and re-watch them as needed.

Here are the results of a quick survey of some STEM and premed students about which study tools they used with success:

Study tools:
Anki
Quizlet
Remnote
Roam
Obsidian
Substrate (www.withsubstrate.com) A video game-based study tool for organic chemistry. Still in beta, and it requires that your professor signs up too.

Note taking Tools:
Notability
GoodNotes
Evernote

Cover the syllabus for each course. Familiarize yourself with the course syllabus. Use your syllabus to prepare ahead for class. This allows you to concentrate on learning and studying rather than feeling lost and searching for meaning during a lecture. I noticed this culture of studying from old exams in medical school (I was probably too young in college to have caught on). The problem, then, is that you are only studying what one professor repeatedly includes on her or his exams. This is why we have all noticed some brilliant friends who did really well in class, turn out a poor performance on national standardized tests. Unlike Arlene, I was not a *brilliant* student, but I always did better on these tests because I learned to study according to a syllabus and from actual textbooks. Today, I know of a few young students who barely ever cracked open a textbook and now have a college degree! That is not going to work in medical school. Cover the syllabus!

Tutors- Immediately seek understanding of a difficult concept or subject with which you are struggling to learn. Do not let anything stumble you for too long. It will just snowball and the subject becomes more difficult. This leads us to another strategy for having a high science GPA- **Get a tutor for each science subject**. Professors usually have office hours during which a student can visit them and get support or explanations for subject matter that eludes them. However, many schools offer free tutoring centers. Also teaching assistants or college seniors may offer tutoring services that are affordable. I recommend getting a tutor. This way, you can set the hours and place that is best for you.

Time management. This final strategy will serve you well throughout your professional and personal life. Time management is your ability to prioritize, organize, plan and problem solve to accomplish your goals within a certain period. This allows you to maximize the use of your time and even reclaim time, which can then be used for other things. You have control over your time instead of time controlling you. You have less stress and better quality of life.

 This is key. In high school, a student could basically get all their studying and homework/assignment done in a night. In college, graduate and post-grad studies there simply will not be enough hours in the day to complete all of this. So, working harder will not accomplish what is needed here; the student must be prepared to **work smarter**. Mastering your time, prioritizing, and scheduling will be the key to working smarter. So, do yourself a favor and take a good time management course. If you prefer an actual app or software to help you with time management, there are many apps and tools available. I love **the Pomodoro method** where you choose your task, set a timer for 25 minutes, work diligently on that task without interruption until the timer goes off. Then take a 5-minute break and start again until task is completed. I use it currently and it works wonders for me. The Pomodoro technique allows for a structured, painless way for you to touch on each task you have planned for the day. That's what I like - even if it's just 15 minutes, you have done some work on a specific subject, task or goal. Of course, as a premed student, you will need to adjust the times slots and the breaks, like the **52/17 rule**. The method is so effective you may be tempted to keep going and not take the recommended breaks. Take the breaks!

 However fast or slow you learn, or whatever your learning style, or whatever tools or tactics you choose to use, the most important factors in performing well academically are **discipline, consistency and perseverance**. These three qualities will help you achieve your academic goals and overcome most problems. Passion and motivation alone are not enough. If they were, we would all accomplish our dreams! Who isn't passionate and motivated to be Beyoncé and physician astronaut Mae Jemison all rolled into one person? Or a Kobe/Elon? New medical students are shocked into realizing this. They understand that it is not smarts that will get them through medical school; the quantity of work is just too overwhelming. They understand that it will take more than intelligence, that it will take discipline, consistency and perseverance. So, while you are in college, work on cultivating these characteristics in yourselves.

Here is what Dr. Arlene said in her soon to be released book on studying in medical school: '... It's more than study, it's diet and biochem, it's soul and spirit, it's family and peace, it's talent and avoidance of grief, it's ***sticktoitiveness***.' Same applies to your premed studies, have balance in your life but stick-to-it.

We will summarize this chapter on academics with a quote from the ever-popular book Eat That Frog by Brian Tracy: **'Refuse to allow a weakness or a lack of ability in any area to hold you back.** *Everything is learnable.* **And what others have learned, you can learn as well.'**

CHAPTER 8 TIMELINES AND TIME MANAGEMENT

Here is a timeline of the path to medical school from college. Your first step in time management should be to have a plan. Here is your battle plan laid out with every step strategically timed. The last chart is a timeline or pathway for an applicant who is applying after graduating college. Print the timeline out and refer to it every month to keep yourself on track.

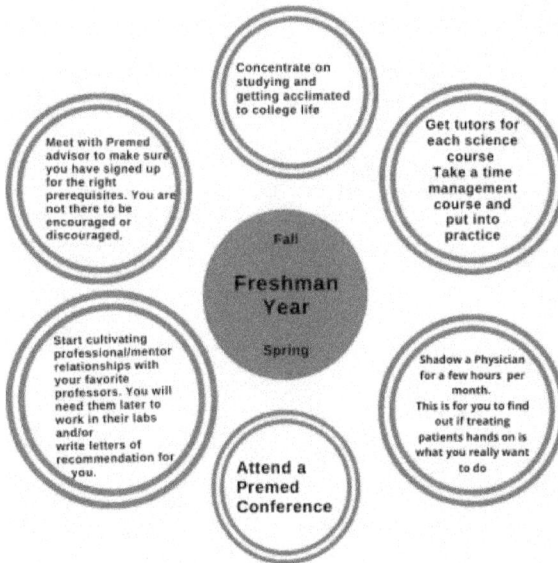

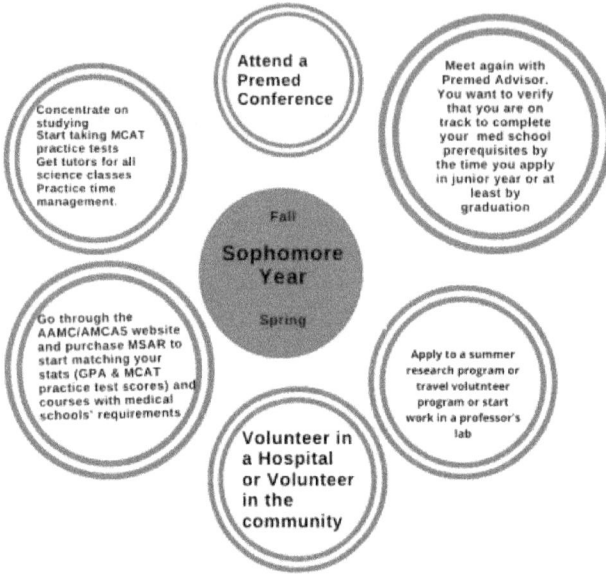

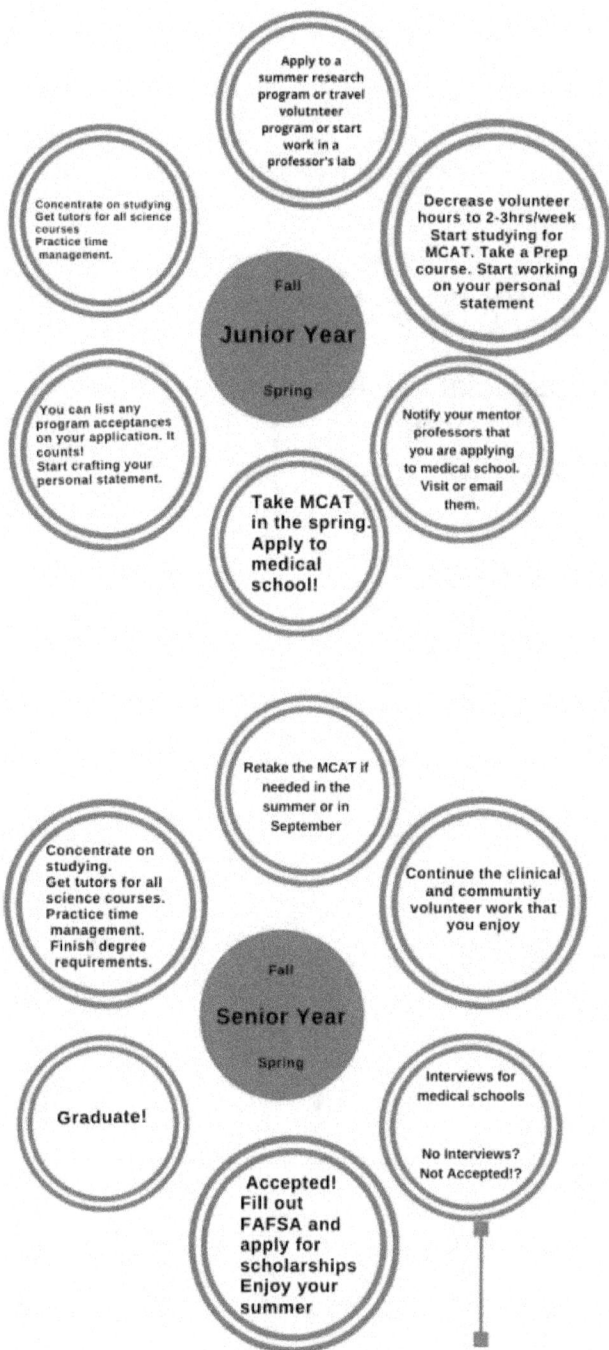

Apply to a summer research program or travel volutnteer program or start work in a professor's lab

Concentrate on studying Get tutors for all science courses Practice time management.

Decrease volunteer hours to 2-3hrs/week Start studying for MCAT. Take a Prep course. Start working on your personal statement

Fall

Junior Year

Spring

You can list any program acceptances on your application. It counts! Start crafting your personal statement.

Notify your mentor professors that you are applying to medical school. Visit or email them.

Take MCAT in the spring. Apply to medical school!

Retake the MCAT if needed in the summer or in September

Concentrate on studying. Get tutors for all science courses. Practice time management. Finish degree requirements.

Continue the clinical and communtiy volunteer work that you enjoy

Fall

Senior Year

Spring

Graduate!

Interviews for medical schools

No Interviews? Not Accepted!?

Accepted! Fill out FAFSA and apply for scholarships Enjoy your summer

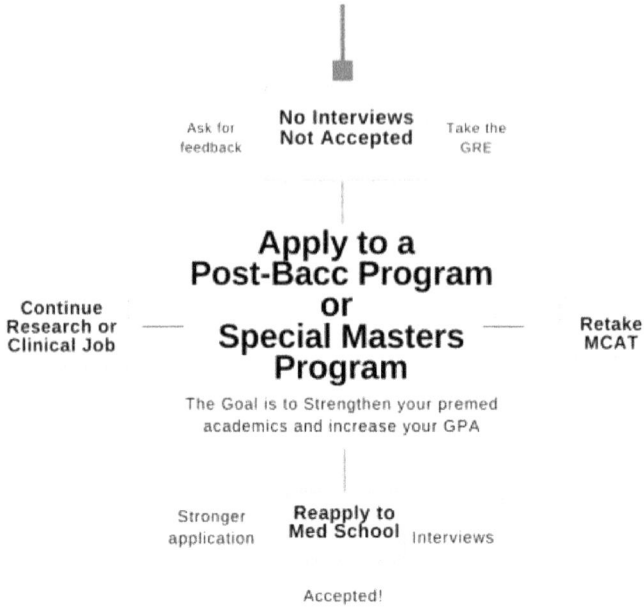

Ask for
feedback

**No Interviews
Not Accepted**

Take the
GRE

Apply to a
Post-Bacc Program
or
Special Masters
Program

Continue
Research or
Clinical Job

Retake
MCAT

The Goal is to Strengthen your premed
academics and increase your GPA

Stronger
application

**Reapply to
Med School**

Interviews

Accepted!

The goal of the book was to prepare you for this moment, so that *you are now a highly qualified candidate for acceptance to medical school*. So, by now you have figured out that this is sort of an exercise in resume building, a resume that you will be presenting to the medical school's admission committee. You are applying for a position; you already have the basic require-ments for the job (good to excellent grades and MCAT scores) and now they are looking to see what sets you apart from the other qualified 'job' candidates. Is your resume interesting enough for you to be granted an interview?

We won't discuss the application process in depth as it is a compilation of everything you have done up to this point. Visit https://students-residents.aamc.org for application in-structions and tips. We will, however, briefly discuss how to choose your medical schools, the MCAT, personal statement, secondary application and the interview process. Your GPA and MCAT score will let the admissions committee know what kind of *student* you will be. However, your narratives (personal state-ment, secondary app essays and interviews) will let them know what kind of *doctor* you will be. As you will see later, you do not have to apply to medical school at a specific time to be ac-cepted. You can and should apply to medical school when you feel your application is strong and when you are emotionally and physically ready.

And the final bit of advice will be mentioned here, first: when you do apply, *Apply Early* in the application cycle! For various reasons, applying early in the cycle increases your chances for acceptance.

How to select medical schools that will maximize

your chances for acceptance

You can use this strategy for other health profession schools. For medical schools you should use the **MSAR** to compare schools' features, policies, requirements, GPA and MCAT scores and more.

For Osteopathic medicine you can use **ChooseDO**, for dental school **ADEA/ AADSAS,** for vet school the **VMSAR**, for physician assistant school **CASPA.**

-Plan to apply to 15 to 20 schools

-Select first your in-state public schools as these will be more favorable to you.

-Select next your in-state private schools. Note what percentage of in-state students they accept. Are there any set asides or preferences? If not whittle down this list.

-Select your regional schools. See which ones give preference to students in the region and add those to the list.

-Now match your medical career goals with the school's goals and mission.

-Go to the individual schools' open house or med school fair if they have one.

-Now select the 15 to 20 schools to which you will apply.

For students who think that their numbers (Science and overall GPA, and MCAT score) are on the lower side but are within the averages you can go further and:

- Dig deeper to find out which schools *immediately* screen out applicants based on GPA and MCAT. Depending on the strength of your numbers you may want to limit applications to these schools. You want an ADCOM to get a chance to look at the rest of your application, and not have some computer algorithm throw out your application due to GPA and MCAT score.

Schools may not be forth coming about their screening policy. Remember, earlier we talked about how many schools will say they do a holistic review of their candidates.

- So, another way to know is to find out which schools are selective about the applicants to whom they will send a secondary application. Again, depending on your numbers, you may want to limit applications to these schools. Apply to schools that automatically send out secondary applications.

THE MCAT

From the AAMC: 'The Medical College Admission Test® (MCAT®) is a standardized, multiple-choice examination designed to assess your problem solving, critical thinking, and knowledge of natural, behavioral, and social science concepts and principles prerequisite to the study of medicine.' It is administered by the AAMC. Many of you have already heard the horror stories of studying for the MCAT. Kill that noise; it's not for you. Review the study techniques discussed in the academic chapter. Most students take the exam in the spring of their junior year, in preparation for applying to medical school that summer. However, you should take this test when you feel that you are well prepared, and that time will be different for some students. As you will see later, you do not have to apply to medical school at a specific time to be accepted. You can and should apply to medical school when you feel your application is strong and when you are emotionally and physically ready.

The exam is a particularly challenging exam. However, in addition to hard, consistent studying, there are a ton of resources and strategies for doing well on the exam. We will mention a few later. First, let's look at what is on the exam.

MCAT SUBJECT CONTENT

The MCAT exam tests a wide range of subjects, such as:
- Organic and inorganic chemistry.
- Physics.
- Biology.
- Biochemistry.
- Basis research methods and statistics.
- Psychology.
- Sociology.
- Ethics, philosophy, cultural studies as well as popula-

tion health, social sciences and humanities.

So how much of each subject do you have to know? The AAMC suggests a year each of general chemistry, organic chemistry, physics, and biology, plus a semester each of psychology, sociology, and biochemistry. On average, students start studying for the exam 6 to 9 months before the test date. The studying is intense and focused, requiring planning and strategy and lots of practice tests. Start with a practice test so that you can assess your strong areas and weak areas. Use the study tools we discussed in the Academics chapter.

Your scores are valid for 2 to 3 years after the exam. Check the policy for each school to which you apply.

In the current version of the MCAT, exam scores are reported in four sections:

- Biological and Biochemical Foundations of Living Systems
- Chemical and Physical Foundations of Biological Systems
- Psychological, Social, and Biological Foundations of Behavior
- Critical Analysis and Reasoning Skills

Most US, Canadian and Caribbean medicals schools require MCAT scores. The MCAT allows for accommodating tests for certain conditions. *Examples of conditions that may qualify for accommodations under the Americans with Disabilities Act (ADA) include, but are not limited to:

- Learning disabilities
- ADHD
- Psychiatric (e.g., depression, anxiety, etc.)
- Sensory impairments (i.e., vision or hearing impairment)
- Physical impairments (e.g., Crohn's disease, pain due

to a physical condition or injury, etc.)

*From AAMC.ORG

MCAT Prep courses – The AAMC offers a ton of support includ-ing study guides, videos, practice tests and more to prepare for the exam. Kaplan MCAT prep, ExamKrackers Mcat, Princeton Review MCAT Review Course, Khan Academy MCAT prep course, The Gold Standard MCAT Prep Course are great prep courses and students can research and compare which prep course is bet-ter for them. However, your student's first introduction to the MCAT shouldn't be their college's mock test in the junior year or a prep course. They should be getting used to the content and format of the MCAT questions in their Freshman and sopho-more years. Often, though, these students have enough stress with their heavy course load and do not like an extra chore put upon them. There are several MCAT prep groups that post ques-tions and answers for free on social media platforms like Insta-gram and Facebook. Since even college students spend time on Instagram, this can become part of that daily IG time and not be so much of a chore.

THE CASPER TEST

The CASPer test is a situational judgement test (SJT) used by academic programs, including some medical schools and physician assistant schools, to help assess applicants for non-academic attributes or people skills. The test consists of 12 sections, video-based and word-based scenarios, with 3 questions that you answer about each scenario over a 60- to 90-minute period. The scenarios are not clinical or academic. This is not a test for which you need to study. This is your chance to show your people skills and judgement abilities. As you go through your premed journey and engage in various medical and clinical settings, observe how experienced doctors, nurses and other clinical staff use discernment, wisdom and empathy to handle patient situations. Even though the test is not clinical based this can help to prepare you for the CASPer test. The test is done online and can be taken in any internet connected location. The results are then sent directly to your selected schools. Check the MSAR to see if your chosen schools require this test. Find out more and take a practice test at: www.takecasper.com

LETTERS OF RECOMMENDATION

Do not be afraid to request a *positive* **letter of recommendation**. For your medical school applications make sure you specifically request a great or glowing recommendation letter from the writer. We have heard numerous medical school admissions committee members state that some recommendation letters are too bland or worse yet, did not even recommend the applicant. It can ruin your chances of being considered for admission. Also, the committee cannot tell you that the recommendation letter was not a good one. We do not know why this happens or why anyone would do this!

We always encourage you to cultivate (professional) relationships with your professors. Besides being a good student, let them know who you are via class, virtual or in-person office hours, emails etc. You will need letters of recommendation for a few things before you need them for medical schools. Maybe start by asking them for an LOR for an activity for which you are applying and include your resume.

Give them something to work with. Also follow up with an in-person thank you or an email thank you note. Many professors expect and welcome you to ask them for letters of recommendation!

THE EXTRACURRICULARS

You get to enter up to 15 experiences. You do not need 15 experiences; a few impactful, consistent activities will be more meaningful than 15 activities that demonstrate no interest or consistency on your part. So, whatever activities you have done, make them count. Show what you learned, how it changed you, how it strengthened your passion and commitment to medicine, and how you contributed. Then review the recommended books in the personal statement section to make sure your copy grabs the attention of the reader and highlights your experiences in the best way.

THE PERSONAL STATEMENT

The Personal Statement is the most powerful *narrative* aspect of your application that can be used to get you the interview that will ultimately get you into medical school. It is your chance to tell the admission committee about:

- Who you are.

- How your experiences have challenged you, and changed you.

- How your experiences fostered your curiosity and passion for medicine.

- Show exactly when, where and how all of this came about.

There are many resources on how to write and format a compelling personal statement. Again, the AAMC shows you how to outline your Personal statement using the allowed 5300 characters (includes spaces). Copywriting 101 from Copyblogger is a great free online resource. It teaches you how to write stories that grab and engage its readers.

Teach the reader something new!

Do show the reader what makes you *unique* from other applicants.

Do get personal and vulnerable. It engages the reader.

Do show the admission committee your soft skills like empathy, compassion, motivation resiliency etc.

Do tell your experiences in the form of stories. *Show* what happened when, and how you were impacted.

Do show *how you impacted* people's lives during your experiences.

Do let everything come together to explain your motivation to become a doctor.

Do let your advisor and others read your essay and critique it.

Don't wait until application season to start writing it, you will be busy with other aspects of the application process and anxious. Start a few months before this, let it develop over the months.

Don't go overboard because when you do get the interview you won't sound like your essay- maybe your humor won't match, your vocabulary won't be consistent with the essay. In other words, please write the essay in a style true to yourself.

Don't try to manipulate the reader with sad stories or gimmicks.

Don't re-list everything on your resume or the extracurriculars section.

Don't discuss poor grades or other deficiencies unless it ties into another story and must be mentioned. You will have other opportunities to explain away poor grades etc.

Don't *fill* your personal statement with a lot of medical or scientific terms. Remember admission committees are made up of not only MDs and PhDs, but PhDs of different fields, ethics professors, counsel, students and academicians of other backgrounds. Write your PS so that any committee member will understand your 'why'.

SECONDARY APPLICATIONS

Secondary applications are applications sent to you directly from the medical school. They are sent to you after the school has received your AMCAS (primary) application. They are specific to that school's goals, mission and requirements. The school gathers further information about you via questions and prompts that require short essay responses. So, this is your time to tell that school how your specific qualities and experiences meet their school's interests and how you can add value to that school. This is also the time to explain away one or two poor grades or other *significant* deficiencies in your application. No application is perfect, therefore resist the temptation to explain away everything you think is deficient. Do not use the same essay for each school's similar questions; don't be like my kids who recycled their Harriet Tubman essay from elementary school all the way through middle school. (I can't believe that worked!). Discern which experiences and qualities you possess that meet a particular school's interests and then discuss those.

A lot of schools do not change their questions on the secondary apps. This provides an opportunity for you to get the questions ahead of time and prepare your answers to them early. This way you are ready to submit them well before the recommended two-week response time frame. The faster you return your secondaries the better, as it shows that you are interested in that particular school and also that you are organized, prepared and serious. However, you must first wait for the schools' prompt to *submit* a secondary app.

Many Schools now automatically send out secondary applications. But there are still some medical schools that only send out secondary apps to a select percentage of students who they have deemed as candidates of interest. You could identify these schools, as a matter of strategy; since these schools obviously have a second round of weeding out candidates for interviews by means of the secondary app, you may or may not want to limit how many of these schools you apply to. Remember secondary apps cost money also!

Remember: **Apply Early!**

THE INTERVIEW

Our goal in this book is to make you a highly qualified candidate for medical school. To make you so interesting that medical schools will want to choose you. Well, there is one last hurdle- the medical school admissions interview. So, you have been granted an interview! You have landed a seat at the table. Congratulations! They have already decided that they want you as a student in their school, but they want to meet you now, talk to you face to face and see what else you have to contribute that may not have been presented on your application. As we mentioned earlier, the interview will allow ADCOMs to see what kind of *doctor* you will be. This is your chance to shine and close the deal. There are now generally three different types of interviews and a school will usually use one or a combination of them:

1.**Traditional one on one interview**. Here you meet with one or more interviewers and you exchange questions.

2. **Multiple Mini Interview**. In this scenario you will meet with several interviewers separately. The interviews are kept short and you move on to the next station to meet with each interviewer until you have met with all of them. MMIs are a relatively new style of interviews that some medical schools have chosen to use. It was first introduced in Canada in 2000. The belief and intent is that the different interviews will reduce bias towards student while also allowing the school to know even more about a student.

3. **VITA**- video interview tool for admissions is offered by the AAMC in response to the limitations imposed by the Covid-19 pandemic. The applicant records a short video answering the question prompts. It is done on your own time, at the request of a school. The AAMC sends you the invitation to create the video, this video is then made available to the other schools to

which you applied upon request.

In any one of these types of interviews, the interviewers may know your scores and application - an **open interview** or they may not- a **blind interview**.

Research the school and its mission before the interview. Be honest about where you stand on ethical issues and why. Be up to date on current major medical developments or discoveries. Be prepared to answer the 'why medicine' question. You will be asked about the positive aspects of your application. However, you may be asked about the negatives; be prepared to eloquently relay your failures, challenges and adversities and how you overcame them (resilience and perseverance). Study your application, especially the personal statement and secondary app essays. You do not want to stumble when questioned about an item on your application. You want to be able to discuss these comfortably if questioned.

Just a quick reminder: for those scenario-based questions that often have no correct answer or conclusion, be mindful that there is a correct *way* that you should be formulating your answer. The interviewer is observing your thought process, problem solving abilities, whether you show empathy, concern and that you understand the importance of teamwork in medicine. There are many resources available to help you sharpen and fine tune your interviewing skills. However, that old, but excellent advice about just being yourself really does apply here. Unlike a job interview where a potential employer is still trying to figure out if you are qualified for the job, by the time you get a medical school interview, you have already been qualified or pre-selected for the position. Now they want to meet you, see what it is like to talk to you, listen to whatever else you have to offer, assess how you will talk to and interact with your future patients! Be that someone to whom people can relate. Show that you can listen and communicate, showing empathy, understanding and kindness. Just be yourself! .....And check out these few resources that we recommend:

www.mockquestions.com

https://www.mockquestions.com/graduateschool/Kansas+City

+University/Medical+School/

Multiple Mini Interview (MMI): Winning Strategies from Admissions Faculty by Samir P. Desa, MD

The Premed Playbook Guide to The Medical School Interview by Ryan Gray, MD

CHAPTER 10 THE NON-TRAD, THE GAP YEAR AND THE REAPPLICANT STUDENTS

Medical schools are reporting that as many as 50% of their newly admitted students were from the group known as **non-traditional students**. Hah! That would make the term a misnomer at this point. Icahn school of Medicine at Mount Sinai New York mentioned that 70% of their incoming students this year had taken at least one **gap year**! Similarly, an admin from UMass said three out of four admitted students had taken a gap year! "Students with post graduate education add to the diversity of our student body. I see this as a positive addition", he said. Finally, some schools report as many as 25% of applications they receive are from **reapplicants**. These statistics reflect the fact that the path to medical school is not always a straightforward one. As I mentioned before with my classmate Jen, there can be zig zags, adjustments and regrouping. Each situation will have its own strategy to successfully gaining acceptance into medical school.

The Gap year student is one who already graduated from college and has completed the medical school prerequisite courses but did not immediately apply to medical school.

The Non-traditional student, as far as medical school admissions go, refers to students who have either: 1-Already graduated from college but did not complete the required pre-medical courses for medical school, or 2- The student who has already had a career and has now decided to pursue a career in medicine.

The Reapplicant student is a student who is re-applying to medical school after being denied acceptance in the previous cycle(s).

Either of these groups of students can do a post-baccalaureate program (post-bacc) or a special masters program (SMP) to complete the required courses, strengthen academic perform- ance and increase chances for admission. Non-traditional stu- dents usually do one of these programs depending on their need. Most students do well in these programs due to a deeper focus and commitment to their goals. These programs are well recognized by medical schools and some medical schools even run these programs.

The post-bacc program is great to complete or retake your pre- requisite courses and raise your GPA. You may want to do this if you finished your degree requirements or graduated but you do not have the required prerequisite courses for medical school. You would then enroll in one of these programs or you can ac- tually put together your own post-bacc program, by re-enroll- ing in college and taking the courses on your own (an informal post-bacc). Students may opt to do the informal post-bacc if they are only missing a few of the required courses and know exactly what is needed. The other reason to do a post-bacc is if you have a *few* courses in which you did not do well and you would like to retake them to raise your *college* GPA. (only a few; you cannot retake all your science courses!) Overall, the post- bacc program can be considered a continuation of college there- fore no additional degree is granted but your college GPA will be adjusted. The goal is to complete your requirements or retake courses, do well in these courses and increase your GPA, thereby strengthening your medical school application and increasing your chances for acceptance.

The SMP, on the other hand, is a one-to-two-year graduate program concentrating in the biomedical sciences and grants a master's degree. You will need to have completed your pre- requisite science courses already, in undergrad, to gain accept- ance to an SMP. Therefore, ***the special masters program is not for those students who need to complete or repeat science pre- requisite courses.*** You will be establishing a graduate GPA; your college GPA will remain as is. Both GPA's will be included in your medical school application. SMP's are usually offered by or affiliated with medical schools and students may be taking classes with medical students. Because of their affiliations with medical schools, SMP's offer more clinical and research experiences along with mentorship. They also prep you along the way for the MCAT exam. SMP's are great to establish another GPA, separate from your college GPA and strengthen your science academics, showing medical schools that you can handle their academics. If you meet their GPA and other requirements in some of these programs you may be guaranteed acceptance into their medical school. These are known as **linked SMP's**.

Sometimes the terms 'post-bacc' and 'SMP' are used interchangeably. Please be careful to determine which program is being offered by a school. Many of the programs list themselves as catering to one or more of the following categories:

Career-changers
Academic record-enhancers
Underrepresented minority students
Economically or educationally disadvantaged students
Accommodates students interested in other health professions

Here is a link to some post-bacc programs compiled by the AAMC: https://apps.aamc.org/postbac/#/index_ You can also see the list in the addendum.

Applying to a post-bacc or SMP can be done on your own, or if you are applying to several schools you may want to simplify the process by using a centralized application service like **PostbacCAS**. According to Liaison, the company who launched the service:

'The Post Baccalaureate Centralized Application Service (PostbacCAS) simplifies the process of applying to post-baccalaureate programs. You start by selecting the programs you wish to apply to, then you submit one application that includes all necessary materials. Once received by PostbacCAS, your application and materials go through a verification process before being transmitted to all of your selected programs.' Here is the link: https://postbaccas.liaisoncas.org/

Please note that not all post-bacc programs participate with this service. Also, note that special masters programs may use different application services.

A **gap year student**, as we previously mentioned, is one who already graduated from college and has completed the medical school prerequisite courses but did not immediately apply to medical school. There may be many valid reasons to take a gap year including simply not being ready, needing a plan to bring your grades up, overwhelmed, having to take care of a sick relative, having mental or physical health issues, or needing to work for an income.

The gap year student differs from the non-traditional student and they need to be strategic about how they use their time. What is different is that the non-trad student would have accomplished meaningful work experience, clinical or research experience organically over the years. A gap year student must be deliberate in showing their continued commitment to medicine during this short time off. You should figure out what activity is the best way for you to do this depending on your circumstances. Applying to one of the post-bacc programs could be the thing to do if poor grades is one of your issues. Perhaps you can use some of the time volunteering in a clinical or community setting a few hours a week. Caring for a sick relative can be viewed as clinical experience as you are actually involved in patient care. If you had to work, demonstrate how your job has taught you new skills or strengthened your desire to pursue medicine even if the job is not medical related. Whatever you are doing during this gap year (or two), show on your application and interviews how you grew during this time, how it prepared you and how it reaffirmed your commitment to a career in medicine.

Reapplicants

Again, the reapplicant student is a student who is re-applying to medical school after being denied acceptance in the previous cycle(s). These students already have met the academic requirements and have taken the MCAT. According to some statistics the national pool of reapplicants is 25%.

Much like the gap year student, a student who is re-applying to medical school after being denied in previous cycle(s) must show a continued commitment to the field of medicine. Most importantly, these students also need to know why they were denied and then develop a plan of action. They can do this by asking the schools for feedback about their application and why they were denied. Some schools may comply with this request while others do not. If none of your schools can give you feedback, re-examine your stats, your application and interview performance yourself, along with your counselors or mentors.

There are numerous reasons why a medical school may deny acceptance to a candidate. We can attempt to address a few of them here.

Poor letters of recommendation. Schools cannot reveal what was said in letters of recommendation submitted on your behalf. A poor letter of recommendation can ruin your chances for acceptance. This is why it is important to ask specifically for a *great* letter of recommendation from your professors and others. This may sound presumptuous but it is a necessary step when requesting LORs unless you know the writer really well. Again, we are not leaving anything to chance, so ask.

Your MCAT score and GPA may not have been competitive enough for a particular school. You may then want to retake the MCAT after a renewed study strategy and several months of study. To address a GPA deficiency, you may decide to retake a couple of science courses if the grades were low via a formal or informal post-bacc. If the grades were just mediocre and do not warrant repeating, then you might want to consider a special masters program. This is a chance to show medical schools, on a higher level now, that you can handle the medical school curriculum. It is also a chance to create a separate but *higher* GPA.

A lack of enough community and clinical volunteer hours or clinical work. This is an easier fix. Figure out which clinical and community activities you are passionate about. Seek out a job or volunteer position and excel at it!

The Personal Statement was underwhelming. This is difficult because it is so subjective, and who will tell you? Have your mentors, counselors, perhaps English professors or journalism majors look over your personal statement. Review the tips for a strong personal statement.

The interview did not go well. Practice, practice, practice. That is the best strategy to undertake for improving your interview skills. Ask your school or mentors if they can do mock interviews with you. There are even online resources that offer mock interviews now. However, there is one important factor going into this- you must know yourself! By that, I mean you must know your application inside out, you must know your why and why not, your strengths and weaknesses, your areas of growth and passions. Some students go into an interview and have forgotten things that they included in their application personal statement and secondary application answers. This creates awkward lapses in the interview. It also gives the impression that you were not prepared or worse- that you may have provided false information.

You were not a good fit with the school's goals. Research the schools' missions again. Did you apply to a school with a mission to place doctors in rural medicine settings but gushed about how you loved working in a big city? Applied to a bunch of out of state public medical schools or worse- did not apply to you own state's medical school? These are just a few of the small missteps that a good candidate may make.

Here is what some medical school admission committee members had to say about students who reapply:

"We see a lot of reapps. In fact, the pool is generally about 25% reapplicants. We always like to see what has changed since the last application. Sometimes people who were unsuccessful in one application immediately reapply the next cycle and nothing has really changed. Does that make sense?"

"if you are reapplying, just make sure to write new essays! Don't copy and paste from the previous application!"

"For re-applicants, we always recommend that they continue to clearly display their interest in medicine and why. Additionally, we recommend that you highlight any new activities, experiences, etc. in your application to show the Admissions committee that you still want to pursue a career in medicine."

Whatever you do please revisit the MSAR and do a deeper comparative analysis of the schools to which you *should* apply. Which school's stat averages do you fall within? Which schools' missions matches your experiences and goals. Which means more to you – attending a specific school or pursuing a specific career (becoming a medical doctor)?

So, to summarize for the reapplicant student: Remember there will be an entire year before you can resubmit another round of applications to medical schools. Besides re-strategizing and correcting, during this time you must show a continual interest in medicine and be able to document and verify it.

CHAPTER 11 FINANCING MEDICAL SCHOOL WHILE BUILDING WEALTH

I remember watching in shock as a friend of mine, who was a year or two into residency, drove down 125thStreet in Harlem, New York City in a beautiful purple Porsche convertible. It stood out like a sore thumb on this busy urban street. My mouth was literally hanging open, I couldn't wave or yell out to him in time, he was gone! How could he afford a car that expensive, while the rest of us were worrying about student loan payments? And then I remembered that he didn't have student loans! He had gone to medical school in his home country where, like many other countries, medical school education is subsidized or free. Not so much for us!

In the USA student loan debt has reached epic proportions. Student loan debt has been documented as a contributor to depression, anxiety, and other mental health issues. The average cost of medical school can range from around $30,000 to over $60,000 per year depending on whether the school is an in-state school, public school or a private school.

* 4 Years of Medical School

How Much Does It Cost?	How Much Do Students Borrow?
Public $255,517	$200,000
Private $337,584	$215,000

Few students can afford to pay the full tuition and fees, most rely on student loans. However, with some research and planning this debt can be reduced or avoided all together. We will address strategies to: 1. Reduce or eliminate the cost of applying to medical school 2. Reduce the cost of attending medical school and 3. Eliminating any debt you may acquire for paying to attend medical school. Some of these strategies can be employed early on, during college and medical school or after medical school; some of these strategies are better executed with the help of family members. The AAMC also has great advice on managing money during and after medical school. Here is a link to some of their webinars on this topic: aamc.org/premedresources. Throughout all of this however, one of the most important things you can do is to improve and protect your credit score. This is not because you are going to go off and finance everything! A high credit score will give you the leverage you need for other future financial transactions as you will see later.

*Source:AAMC 2019 Debt, Cost and Loan Repayment Fact Card

THE COST OF APPLYING TO MEDICAL SCHOOL

First let us talk about the *cost of applying to medical school!* Applying to med school is not cheap. The costs for application fees and travel add up very quickly. You should start saving for these costs as soon as you can. See the chart below for a breakdown of these costs as per the AAMC.

Application Expenses	Estimated Range
MCAT Prep Course	$300-2000
MCAT Registration	$320
MSAR	$28
Transcripts	$5-10
Primary Applications (20 Schools)	$930
Secondary Applications ($0-150/ school	$1200
CASPer Exam	$30-60
Interviews (travel, hotel, clothes)	$400-2000

The fee assistance program (FAP) described in the abbreviations-to-know section can eliminate some of these costs for those who qualify. The benefits of the FAP program if you qualify are:

- MCAT official prep products

-Reduced MCAT registration fee from $320 to $130

-MSAR complimentary subscription

- Waiver or all AMCAS fees for 1 application with up to 20 med school designations

These benefits can save you up to $2000 or more. There are other ways to fund the application cost if needed. One pre-health advisor at the AAMC medical school virtual fair came up with an interesting plan: instead of Christmas and birthday gifts from relatives, ask each relative for money for the application fee for one school and then, associated costs if you get an interview. We love this idea! For those of you looking for other ideas see the end of this chapter for resources to save and grow money painlessly starting now!

Many students do not realize that there are scholarships available on the graduate level. I know of an engineering student who did a master's in engineering, paid for solely by scholarships! The scholarships available for medical school can be offered by the institution (including tuition free schools), service based or private organizations or corporations.

Tuition free schools - We can start with this dream scenario first; it is available and possible after all. By now, everyone has heard about the wonderful announcement from NYU that tuition would be free to their medical students. There are a few medical schools that pioneered this and others that soon followed. These tuition free programs vary in exactly what is free and for whom it is free. For example, Columbia University's scholarship is for need-based students while UCLA's covers all students plus living expenses. Do your research. Here is a list of tuition free medical schools. It may not be complete as the number of schools is slowly growing:

1. **New York University School of Medicine**

2. **Weill Cornell Medical College**

3. **Cleveland Clinic Lerner College of Medicine – Case Western Reserve University**

4. **Washington University School of Medicine**

5. **Kaiser Permanente School of Medicine (temporary)**

6. **UCLA David Geffen**

7. **Columbia University Vagelos College of Physicians and Surgeons**

One of the reasons medical schools offer free tuition is to encourage students to go into primary care. Many students feel they must pursue higher paying specialties to be able to afford to pay back their student loans and have money left over for a decent life. For many, these higher paying specialties are not their passion or first choice. It creates undue stress and competition among medical students. Eliminating their heavy student loan debt will allow students to pursue and concentrate on the specialty that they actually want. The hope is that this will increase the number of students going into primary care. Some schools want to encourage students to go into rural medicine.

MD/PhD Programs – Many of these medical scientist training programs are tuition free. These are highly competitive and intensive programs. So, we mention this as a matter of knowledge for you highly motivated students who have chosen this path. Applying to these programs only because they are tuition free is not advised and strongly discouraged. See a list of programs at the end of the book.

Scholarships and Grants – There are many scholarships available for health professions students including medical students. There are scholarships for students who commit to working in underserved or rural areas and then there are scholarships available for the Zombie Apocalypse! Students must do their research because there are always new scholarships being added or requirements changing. Scholarships can be institutional, service based or private. Use search engines like Scholly, Unigo or Fastweb. Their websites and apps allow you to enter specific details about yourself and your interests and then match you with scholarship opportunities based on that. The Scholly app is great in that it is working for you all the time and notifies you when matches are found. Also, Scholly offers a free math problem solver and a free writing assistant, an editor for your essays, papers etc. They also sponsor their own scholarships in collaboration with other companies. There are other scholarship search sites. So, money for medical school is out there. Search far and wide but also search near and niched!

Institution Based Scholarships - Many schools offer their own scholarships through endowments or donations. Some of the scholarships are small. Other schools, like Morehouse School of Medicine which offers a $100,000 scholarship to each student, have scholarships that can *greatly* offset the cost of attending.

Service Based Scholarships - These scholarships are usually offered by the military and the federal or state government. The scholarship is granted with stipulations like service in the military for a specific number of years or practicing in underserved areas for a specific time. Here is a partial list of these scholarship-offering programs:

National Health Service Corps Scholarship

Health Professions Scholarship Program (HPSP) – The Army, Navy and Air Force offer a service scholarship to students who attend medical and dental school programs. Students receive full tuition and fee coverage as well as reimbursement of health insurance costs and other school related expenses.

NIH – Medical Research scholars' scholarship

ROTC – The health professions scholarship provides full tuition and a monthly stipend.

Private Scholarships - These types of scholarships are offered by corporations or private organizations. They are sometimes overlooked because people tend to focus on the better-known government scholarships.

National Medical Fellowships – This organization's mission is to build the next generation of healthcare leaders. It offers numerous scholarships to underrepresented minority students. www.nmfonline.org

Chinese American Physicians Society (CAPS) – The student does not have to be Asian.

Vietnamese American Medical Association

American medical Association Physicians of Tomorrow -This is for 3rd year medical students and it awards $10,000 each year.

Pisacano Scholars Leadership Program -This is for 3rd year medical students who demonstrate a 'strong commitment to the specialty of family medicine' and it awards $7,000 each year up to $28000 maximum. www.pisacano.org

Achievement Rewards for College Scientists (ARCS) www.arcsfoundation.org

This is just an example of the diversity of scholarships that are out there for medical school.

See the AAMC list of scholarships. Also, @theprettymed has an excellent list of medical school scholarships done by categories on her website.

Eliminating Medical School Student Loan Debt

There majority of students take out student loans to finance their education. There are programs and strategies to reduce the amount of debt owed or to pay it back faster.

Loan Repayment Programs – Loan repayment programs either forgive your debt after you have made a certain number of payments or they forgive or reduce the debt if you work in certain areas or specialties. This is not you shirking your responsibility to pay back your loans. This is you trading your gifts, talents and time in exchange for the debt reduction. A barter. Some programs are listed below:

PSLF Public Service Loan Forgiveness- This program forgives Direct student loans balances after you have made 120 payments while working for a qualified employer. Here is the link for more information: https://studentaid.gov/manage-loans/forgiveness-cancellation/public-service

NHSC Loan Repayment Program

NIH Loan Repayment Program – 'Since tomorrow's medical breakthroughs will be made by investigators starting in their research careers today, the LRPs represent an important investment by NIH in the future of health discovery and the wellbeing of the Nation'.

EDRP- The VA's Education Debt Reduction Program (EDRP) provides up to $40,000 a year — or $200,000 over a five-year period — in loan repayment. Your commitment is a five-year employment at the Veterans Health Administration. You can leave before the five years are up, but your repayment will be adjusted.

The Federal Student Loan Repayment Program- www.opm.gov

The US Military Health Profession Loan Repayment Program

Note: Some students combine the loan forgiveness and loan repayment programs and max out   the benefits.

Shared Harvest Fund - The Shared Harvest Fund was founded by 3 medical doctors who understood the pain of having student loan debt and the mental anguish it can cause.

The idea was that a student, postgrad or professional could volunteer for a cause and at the same time reduce student loan debt. Volunteer for a project that matches your skill set and, upon completion, the fund pays $200-$1000 directly to your student loan servicer! Then you can repeat the process with different projects until your loan is paid down. Visit www.sharedharvestfund.org to find out more.

Refinancing your student loans is an option. It saves you interest and lowers your payments. However, the lower payments are not the goal. You may have to raise your payment amount to cover the interest. You want out race that new lower interest rate. Otherwise, it defeats our purpose here.

Also, refinancing excludes you from the Public Service Loan Forgiveness program and income-driven repayments. So be ready to give these up.

BE YOUR OWN BANK

College Savings Plan – Parents you can start a 529 College Savings Plan. There are dozens of these plans and different types, savings or prepaid, in-state or out of-state, individual or custodial. Choose one that is of benefit to you and your student. Some financial advisors do not like these plans as they will reduce the amount of need-based financial aid, others say it is never too late to open a plan for your student. If you can fully fund it to cover the entire cost of college and or medical school, it will not matter. Consult with your advisor before opening one.

Note: Consider grandparents to fund these. The plan will not reduce financial aid eligibility this way.

You can also make it fun by choosing a plan that offers Ugift crowdfunding. Much like the plan we talked about for paying for application costs, this allows friends and family to contribute at any time to your
529 College Savings Plan. The plan gives you your own 'crowdfunding page' and you can personalize it, share the code on social media and invite contributors.

Roth IRA – This is a retirement account that you can contribute a capped amount each year. However, you can withdraw funds for education tax free. Also, these accounts do not reduce the amount of need based financial aid for which your student could qualify. You may want to contribute to these first, then the 529 College Savings Plan.

Stocks- Investing in stocks or other financial instruments is an excellent way to save for medical school. Start early enough and you could possibly pay for a significant portion of medical school. (You would not want to use all of your investments.) If you are off to a later start, look forward to paying down your loans faster. Either way, you are engaging in that most important financial principle by making your money work for you! Start to enjoy that feeling of watching your money work and grow. Educate yourself on dividend stocks. Many people are afraid of investing in stocks; however, historically, the stock market has always performed well over a long-term period.

Here are some apps that students can start using today to buy stocks:

Stash

Robinhood

Acorn - one of their cool features is it rounds up your change from credit/debit card purchase and invests the change in fractional shares of stocks.

Later, when you feel comfortable with investing you can open a full(er) brokerage account like

TD AmeriTrade or E*Trade or others.

Jobs - Some people have been known to work their way through medical school and pay for their tuition/room and board. This is not recommended but it is necessary for some students.

We do recommend Danielle Pierce's book on side hustles Baby Steps to Financial Freedom in which she discusses 30 quick-start income-producing side hustles.

Passive income - from Instagram, Facebook, ebooks, courses, services. Many of you have massive social media followings and can monetize them with these digital products and influencing.

After Medical School

Length of Residency	3 years
Student Loans	$200,000
Residency Salary	$60,000
Post-Residency Salary or Income	$190,000

When you break down the student loan amount vs your future income starting with residency, you can face it head on. Depending on who you are, it may not be as overwhelming to pay back medical school loans as you once thought. During residency, if you live on the same income as you lived on during college, you might be able to start paying some of the interest down to keep the loan amount as close to the principal as possible. Then post-residency, when you are making a six-figure salary, if you lived on your resident's salary you may be able to pay off these loans in 3-4 years! (5-6 years if you have undergraduate loans). This takes discipline. We recommend reading the ever popular The White Coat Investor by James M. Dahle, MD.

The next 3 suggestions can allow you to acquire assets and build equity faster. As a doctor you may have a heavier student loan debt, but you can use your income and good credit to your advantage.

Physician Home loan – This is a mortgage for physicians that allows a small down payment but no private mortgage insurance (PMI)

203K fixer upper home loans - This is a mortgage with renovation funds included in the loan. With careful renovation planning, this can create immediate equity in your home.

Tax Lien and Tax Deed Properties - This is my absolute favorite way to build wealth, gain immediate equity and, potentially, rental income. It does not require down-payments nor income or credit checks. We learned how to purchase tax lien and tax deed properties from the great Danielle Pierce, founder of the Real Estate Profit Lab. I wish I knew of this when I was in school. This tax lien properties strategy is best done with family or a spouse/partner involved as it will require other duties and responsibilities, but well worth it.

Tax lien properties can be acquired for as little as $500 in some parts of the country. What if you won at least one of these properties at auction each semester and the actual market value of the property is $40,000-50,000? That is $80,000 - 100,000 worth of property that you will acquire each year that can offset the cost of college and medical school. Now what if these properties were rental properties? That is a passive income stream that, technically, you could use to pay your student loans each month. Or what if you later sold *some* of the properties to completely pay off your student loans at the end of residency when the loans become due? What if you started buying these properties starting in college and sold some of the properties to pay for medical school? The possibilities and scenarios are numerous, but each will provide a way for you to pay for your education while building wealth.

CHAPTER 12 **THE COVID PIVOT**

Love in the time of Covid. (Yes, we tried it too.) An ode to one of our favorite books- Love in The Time of Cholera by Gabriel Garcia Marquez. Unlike the double meaning of the title and the epidemic of that period, we are living through an actual *pandemic* caused by the SARS CoV 2 virus. However, much like the time in the novel, people are still going about their lives- falling in love, getting married (or not), having babies, and still trying to get into medical school! In fact, the AAMC reports an increase of 17% in the number of medical school applications received so far this cycle. One school saw a 35% increase!

So, yes, you still have to do the work. Medical schools have given no indication that they will be reducing their academic or non-academic requirements for acceptance into medical school. Even if they did, please remember that there are still only but so many seats in any one medical school. That has not changed… yet. One adcom went so far as to point out that if current health care workers are risking their lives during this pandemic to continue delivering high quality care to their patients, then why can't you show the same commitment, why should med schools lower their standards?

So, with schools and research labs and summer programs shut down or limited to online, how do you complete your academic and non- academic activities that will get you into medical school? Like many businesses that continued to thrive during this pandemic, you will have to pivot and adjust. This chapter is about some of the pivots we learned going through the premed process with one family member and from our followers @themedicalschoolstrategist.

By now you are well familiar and experienced with online classes and are hopefully adjusted and doing well in your courses. Hopefully, you guys took advantage of your professors' virtual office hours. Now is also a good time to send a 'hello' email to your supervisors, PI's or a professor who knows you, etc. just checking in on them during this pandemic. This a great way to stay in touch now that we are all working or learning remotely. If you are comfortable, include an email profile pic or a photo signature as a reminder of who you are. Hey, we have to find new ways to build and maintain relationships now. You will need these relationships for letters of recommendation later for internships, summer programs and then for your medical school applications. For requests to professors to join a lab or write a letter of recommendation, see the templates at the end of the book.

It is also important to keep networking with other professionals or student colleagues. Keep your social media and LinkedIn current. If you do not have a LinkedIn account, create one now.

Over the last few months, we have seen some of the programs we discussed earlier move to a virtual format. Loop Abroad and FIMRC for example have online projects in which you can participate. NASA's fall internship is online this year. Did we mention that they have great paid internships for premed and STEM students? Apply for spring and summer internship now at intern.nasa.gov.

Physician shadowing: There are still opportunities to shadow physicians but if your state still has restrictions due to the pandemic there are virtual options. See if your school's pre-health department has a database of physicians to shadow via Zoom or Skype or whatever. Many schools do. There are also new resources dedicated to helping students gain those physician shadowing hours:

www.webshadowers.org

www.virtualshadowing.com

https://www.prehealthshadowing.com

You can get a few hours of experience every week. You also have the option to take a short assessment at the end and receive a certificate of attendance. I would recommend that you take that option as this officially documents your hours.

Research: Due to the Covid-19 pandemic many university research programs have been closed to students as part of the safety measures. Other institutions have students participating in online research. Students have been encouraged to concentrate on scientific research procedures, protocols, statistics. One method of scientific research that can be conducted online is **Meta-Analysis**. A meta-analysis is a statistical analysis that combines the results of multiple scientific studies. Meta-analysis can be performed when there are multiple scientific studies of the same subject, compare the data for similarities or variations. The method used is objective statistical data (as opposed to subjective narrative). One scientist told us that she has her students use **The Cancer Atlas Genome** (TCGA). Researchers and students can access the data portal and download cancer data for analysis. If you are new to research, ask a professor for other resources and assistance.

 https://www.cancer.gov/about-nci/organization/ccg/ research/structural-genomics/tcga

https://portal.gdc.cancer.gov/

Here are other sources where you can create your own or join research projects or case studies, access instrumentation and other resources:

www.learngala.com

http://nano4me.org/

www.scistarter.org

NCBI-BLAST

www.jove.com A scientific video journal! You can self-learn some lab procedures.

Here are some impactful activities in which premeds can participate:

1. **Donate blood or organize a blood drive** - One of the fallouts of the Covid-19 pandemic is blood bank shortages around the country. Healthy students can donate or help organize a blood drive.
2. **Educate** - Premed students can use their scientific background to help correct misinformation and myths about the Covid-19 virus - Learn and then educate others about the CDC guidelines for this pandemic. You can do this through social media or write a short article for your local newspaper

or neighborhood newsletter.

3. **Volunteer** – Here are some sites to check out volunteer opportunities:

   www.volunteermatch.org

   www.allforgood.org

   www.pointsoflight.org

   www.idealist.org

   www.hfny.org Hope for New York has a great many virtual volunteer opportunities

   and, also urgent needs opportunities.

   www.crisistextline.org/become-a-volunteer/ According to the Mental Health Fund the mental health impact of Covid-19 will outlast the virus. The Crisis Text Line trains volunteers to support people during the crisis.

   www.physiocamp.org An online volunteer opportunity to teach or tutor K-12 students on health care or medical related topics.

4. **Virtual scribe** - Virtual medical scribes are not new of course. However, some healthcare facilities are employing virtual scribes to fill the increasing documentation caused by recent surges in patient encounters due to Covid-19.

With a loss of employees and increased burden on healthcare workers due to the coronavirus pandemic, medical scribes fill an even more important role. I know of one premed student scribe who lost her job at her urgent care facility due to the lockdown but found work as a virtual scribe.

There are many medical scribe companies but here are 3 that we recommend –

Proscribemd.com

ScribeAmerica.com

Scribekick.com

All of these companies have their own training program to become a medical scribe or they can hire you directly as an experienced scribe. (you could check with **medicalscribe.org** if you want to train on your own. But why pay?) Either way the training is not long, 1- 4 weeks depending on which company you go with. Some of the companies pay during the training period. Be prepared to pass a typing speed test when you sign up.

ProscribeMd and ScribeAmerica seem to be popular among students but I really liked Proscribe's benefits. They are specifically for premed students: letters of recommendation for med school, MCAT Kaplan course scholarships, mock interview at Ross University School of Medicine and coaching. We spoke to one of their directors who confirmed these benefits.

5. **Contact Tracer** – To get a job as a contact tracer, you must first complete a short training course like the one offered by John Hopkins University and receive a certificate of completion. Enroll here: https://www.coursera.org/learn/covid-19-contact-tracing

This job may be more suitable to students who already have healthcare work experience.

6. **myCovidMD** - Created by The Shared Harvest Fund which we mentioned in the finance chapter, this part of their organization was created to 'answer the Call to Action and provide virtual triaging, home testing and more' to fight the covid-19 pandemic. Visit www.mycovidmd.app to sign up to volunteer.

Changes in the MCAT

Covid-19 pandemic has also affected exam dates for the MCAT and how the exam will be administered. After an initial panic and disappointment many students have pivoted, using the postponement of exam dates to study more for the exam. Others have delayed taking the exam since there are now later test dates. Here is what the AAMC has to say about Covid-19 MCAT changes: 'A shortened exam will be administered to accommodate three test appointment times per test date at test centers. The exam time will be reduced from a total "seated" time of 7 hours and 30 minutes to 5 hours and 45 minutes. The number of scored questions remains the same. Other elements of the exam have been reduced or removed to shorten the seated time. Content on the Shortened MCAT Exam Students will still be tested on all four sections of the exam and will be responsible for demonstrating the same knowledge and skills at the same levels of difficulty as on the full-length exam.'

CHANGES IN INTERVIEW TYPE

Other than the location (virtual), interviews remain the same with one new added tool. The VITA- video interview tool for admissions is offered by the AAMC in response to the limitations imposed by the Covid-19 pandemic. The applicant records a short video answering the question prompts. It is done on your own time, at the request of a school. The AAMC sends you the invitation to create the video, this video is then made available to the other schools to which you applied upon request. The VITA does not replace the other types of interviews; it is done in addition to them.

3 Quick Virtual Interview Tips:

- Get dressed. Seems obvious right? However, some people may be tempted to dress the part only from the waist up. Please don't! Be comfortable, but dress professionally from head to toe.

- Look into the camera and not at the screen. When we look at someone on our screens we tend to look down.

- Have some questions ready to ask your interviewer. It shows interest and gives you a little time to relax and regroup.

So, let's summarize:

- You want to go to medical school and become a doctor.
- You need to do very well in your premed courses. So, you'll find your best learning habits and tools, be disciplined, get tutors for each science course, attend tutoring, come up with a **study schedule** and stick to it as much as possible.
- You will be **conscious of your spiritual and emotional needs**. You will put aside time for family, friends, fun and exercise. You will be as disciplined with these things as you are with your studies.
- You will **cultivate student mentor relationships** with your professors. You need academic help and mentorship from them, and they need to know you so that they can write *great* letters of recommendation for you.
- You will participate in **research, jobs and activities** that show your commitment to the field of medicine.
- You will consistently work on a **passion project** that makes you and your application stand out and be memorable!
- You will **start studying for your MCAT exam several months before the exam** and take a prep course.
- You will apply to medical school when you feel ready. You will **apply early in the application cycle**.
- **You will be accepted to medical school!**
- Rinse and repeat (research, volunteer, work, high USMLE scores etc.) to **get the residency you want** and become the doctor in the specialty you truly desire!

Remember: Check your inbox, spam and *special promotions* folders! You do not want to miss out on important updates, deadlines or requests for further information and missing documents from AMCAS or the medical school.

There may be sickness and depression and weariness and break ups and broken hearts along the way, but you just keep moving forward. Just like you take your next step, you take your next course. Just like you take your next breath, you take your next exam. You keep moving forward.

"Never give up on a dream just because of the time it will take to accomplish it. The time will pass anyway." Earl Nightingale Enjoy the journey!

CHAPTER 14 **CONCLUSION**

I remember one day sending my pre-vet daughter a message stating GET ON A BUS NOW! I followed up with a phone call explaining why: A whale had washed up on the beach near our home in the Northeast. Never had this happened in our area. The whale was unfortunately dead and there was to be a necropsy. A necropsy! 5 minutes from our house was the opportunity of a lifetime for her. Or so I thought at the time. In my mind, she should get here asap, approach those in charge, explain that she was a pre-vet student who was interested in helping in anyway in this great undertaking. They would say yes, and she would have participated in the necropsy of a whale. Now which vet school could turn her down?! She promptly shut down my entire scheme with a solid NO. No, she would not get on the bus, no she was not going to try to participate in this serious matter, no. Well at the time I was upset but I can laugh now and appreciate her discernment as to whether advice was hysterical or helpful. She accepted guidance, but she did things her own way and in the end, she was accepted to two vet schools.

In the end be yourself, meaning- choose from the activities that we have listed here but choose something that is enjoyable and challenging to you, something that makes you happy. Look upon the advice and suggestions from parents and others as guidance as to where you should be on this path to medical school, not instructions.

Please do what makes you happy. I had one daughter who did the STEPUP research program with the National Institute of Health when in high school. By college, she was not interested in any STEM careers. (Although the experience features prominently on her resume). My other daughter was also privileged with acceptance into this program in the summer of her junior year of high school. However, she was also accepted into APSA China. My heart stopped when she chose to go to China for 6 weeks instead of the paid NIH research position. By college she was a pre-vet student who did research for two years. Today she is in Vet school. She reminds me now, whenever I make suggestions about school, that her final choices have worked well for her. So, humble brags aside, fear not students and parents: there is more than one play within the battle plan. Students: follow the plan that we have laid out. Accomplish each objective that we have discussed but ***do it in a way that is enjoyable and fulfilling to you***. Within each objective there are many choices, so pick a program or institution or location that is motivating and of interest to you.

I looked around at my medical school classmates on graduation day as we sat in a hall at Lincoln Center NYC. I shuddered at what I saw. I personally knew that some of the guys were still throwing spitballs, were chewing and spitting tobacco and other unmentionables. They probably looked at me and shuddered too! I was a 24-year-old naive fool. But we all had a deep passion and eagerness for our profession and had received a great education. We would go on to have great, fulfilling careers. This is a noble profession but a very humbling one. I feel that what people see as arrogance in doctors is, actually, a weariness and an acceptance of this force called life. As a doctor you will see the absolute highs of medicine and the absolute lows. Successes and failures. You will be an 'untrained research scientist' as you assess what works and what does not work, all within the confines of First Do No Harm. You will make medical discoveries. The grace is that the failures and the lows are far outnumbered by the discoveries, the successes and the highs. Welcome!

It's a beautiful spring day, much like the one at the beginning of this book. You change into your scrubs, grab your stethoscope and stop for your favorite iced coffee. You walk from campus to the medical center. An exciting day in Peds clinic awaits you. You enter the facility and someone yells "Good afternoon doctor!" It seems like it was directed at you, but you look around in puzzlement. It's you! That's you in a few months – a student doctor!

ABOUT THE AUTHORS

Dr Patricia Ann Nowell-Twum is a podiatrist who has practiced for over twenty years in New York. As an undergraduate, she attended Medgar Evers College, CUNY and received a BS in Biology. Dr. Twum attended the New York College of Podiatric Medicine and later completed her residency at Metropolitan Hospital in NYC. She worked for several years at Mount Sinai Morningside Hospital (formerly St. Luke's Roosevelt) and is currently in private practice. She lives in Queens, New York with her husband and family.

Dr. Arlene Blake-McCain is a bilingual physician who practices family medicine. Dr. Blake-McCain attended University of The West Indies Mona and has a BSc in Biochemistry. She attended medical school at Institute of Superior Medical Sciences Havana Cuba, Faculty of Medical Sciences. She also has extensive postgraduate medical experience from her residency in Anesthesia and Intensive Care at UWI Mona. She completed an observership at Piedmont Athens Regional Hospital in Athens, Georgia. She is a former teaching fellow at St. George's University School of Medicine where she taught medical students. Dr. Blake-McCain currently enjoys seeing patients in her private practice in Kingston, Jamaica. She lives in Jamaica with her husband and daughter and is an avid dreamer. :)

Via @themedicalschoolstrategist, Dr Ann and Dr. Arlene have counseled and encouraged hundreds of students throughout their premed journey. Follow us on Instagram and Facebook for current premed strategies and events! Also, email us for continued support and advice at info@themedicalschoolstrategist.com
We hope you enjoyed the book! If so, kindly leave a review on the purchase site. Also, if you have friends and family who

may find value in this book, please share the purchase link with them.

ACKNOWLEDGEMENTS

Thank you to Kam, Kris, Richie, Kearon and Dwight for your input and enthusiastic survey responses. You provided the Millennial/Gen Z insight the book needed. To Monica Aspra Rubi, thank you for your early review and sharing your premed journey with us. (Congrats to Richie and Monica on your recent acceptance to medical school!) Thank you Kamilah Nowell for the cover design and editing. Thank you Cici 'the Six Figure Chick' Gunn who provided knowledge, inspiration and motivation freely to thousands of us who never knew we had a book in us. Sleep in peace Cici.

Please note that the following lists of research programs, BS/
MD programs, post-bacc programs and MD/PhD programs are
by no means complete. The links on some programs may be
old but you can research the program by name. Also, with the
current pandemic there are sure to be changes and updates.
We encourage anyone with new information to email us at
info@themedicalschoolstrategist.com.

SHPEP Programs www.shpep.org

SHPEP is implemented at 12 universities across the nation. Each institution provides scholars with academic enrichment in the basic sciences and math, clinical experiences, career development activities, learning and study skills seminars, and a financial planning workshop. Program sites vary on how they deliver each of these required components and their program start date.

Columbia University

SHPEP at Columbia University Irving Medical Center provides students interested in pursuing a career within the health professions with a well-defined, integrated approach to learning, focusing on the core science curriculum needed to apply to health professions schools for medicine, dentistry, nursing, physical therapy, public health, nutrition, and occupational therapy.

Howard University

SHPEP at Howard University is committed to providing an outstanding academically enriched program that is intended to contribute to a culture of health and promote diversity in health care by strengthening the academic proficiency and team-based care approach of underrepresented minority and disadvantaged students interested in pursuing careers in the health sciences.

Rutgers, The State University of New Jersey

This innovative program will cultivate the interprofessional leaders of tomorrow who have the knowledge, skills and attitude to impact the health and healthcare of our communities. The Summer Health Professions Education Program encompasses Rutgers New Jersey Medical School, School of Dental Medicine, School of Nursing and Ernest Mario School Pharmacy.

University of Alabama at Birmingham

The Summer Health Professions Education Program is a partnership between the University of Alabama at Birmingham (UAB) School of Medicine (SOM), School of Dentistry (SOD), School of Optometry (SOO), and School of Health Professions (SHP), home to the Physician Assistant program. The program goal is to increase diversity in health professions by recruiting and preparing underrepresented students.

University of California Los Angeles and Charles R. Drew University

At the UCLA/ CDU SHPEP, we are committed to developing future leaders that will change the face of medicine, dentistry and nursing as well as to improve health care delivery, policy and research in underserved communities.

University of Florida

UF SHPEP is an immersive program where scholars will engage in case-based learning and interprofessional experiences. Scholars will learn to prepare for the rigors of professional school through our academic program and workshops on successful study strategies. The University of Florida Health Science Center (UFHSC) houses six health related colleges (Dentistry, Medicine, Nursing, Pharmacy, Public Health & Health Professions, and Veterinary Medicine).

University of Iowa

The University of Iowa Health Sciences Colleges are pleased to offer an enriching six-week experience with SHPEP. The Health Sciences Colleges include the Carver College of Medicine, College of Dentistry, College of Pharmacy, and College of Public Health. We strongly believe in the value of exposing students from underrepresented backgrounds to the possibility of pursuing health fields and supporting their goals in accomplishing that dream to help improve the health of society at large.

University of Louisville

"Shaping the Future of Dentistry, Medicine, Nursing and Pharmacy"
The Summer Health Professions Education Program (SHPEP) at the

University of Louisville, introduces prospective medical, dental, nursing, and pharmacy scholars to the academic rigors of health professions education.

University of Nebraska

The Summer Health Professions Education Program (SHPEP) at the University Nebraska Medical Center (UNMC) offers a dynamic and interdisciplinary academic enrichment experience that emphasizes a global approach to learning. Our cross-cutting interprofessional curriculum is comprised of faculty and staff from the UNMC Colleges of Medicine, Dentistry, Nursing, Public Health, and Allied Health Professions (Physical Therapy

University of Texas Health Science Center at Houston

UTHealth is an academic health center that educates more than 5,000 professionals each year, and that delivers health care to patients with diverse cultures, beliefs and nationalities. UTHealth is committed to creating an environment that values inclusion, collaboration, partnerships and teamwork to accomplish its mission.

University of Washington

The UW SHPEP will emphasize a culture of health by encouraging scholars to consider from the cellular to the global level factors that influence health. In addition, scholars will be encouraged to explore what their unique role will be in improving the health of communities with curricula exploring self-identity, culture and personal strengths in a context presenting a range of health professions. Rigorous academic course work will include population health, life sciences, and biostatistics and will utilize lectures, active learning, discussions, peer mentoring and self-reflection.

Western University of Health Sciences

The WesternU Summer Health Professions Education Program offers an innovative approach to academic enrichment in basic sciences through team-based learning. WesternU SHPEP is a rigorously interprofessional program offered in a diverse and vibrant urban environment. Student learning of foundational science, inter-professional teamwork, health disparities, and healthcare policy will be driven by weekly clinical cases.

Other Programs around the country
https://www.joslin.org/research/learning-training-joslin/
summer-student-research-internship

https://www.upstate.edu/grad/programs/summer.php

The National Science Foundation funds research projects in many schools around the country   https://www.nsf.gov/crssprgm/reu/list_result.jsp?unitid=5047

Programs with Many Opportunities in Biology

- The Leadership Alliance, Summer Research – Early Identification Program (SR-EIP)

- National Aeronautics and Space Administration (NASA) OSSI

- Oak Ridge National Laboratories (ORNL), Oakridge, TN: *multiple opportunities in biology and other fields, multiple deadlines, first deadline January 15.*

- University of Oregon: *no hard deadline.*

Programs Emphasizing Ecology / Evolution / Plants / Animals

- American Museum of Natural History (evolutionary biology)

- American Society of Plant Biologists (ASPB)

- Bigelow Laboratory for Ocean Sciences

- California Academy of Sciences, San Francisco, Summer Systematics Institute

- Cary Institute of Ecosystem Studies

. Center for Environmental Research and Conservation, Earth Institute, Columbia University: *Field research in NYC and outside of the continental U.S., applications accepted on a rolling basis.*

. Cornell University and Boyce Thompson Institute for Plant Research, Plant Genome Research Program (PGRG): *Applications due February 7.*

. Cornell University, New York State Agricultural Experiment Station, Geneva, New York

. Donald Danforth Plant Science Center: *applications due February 5.*

. Duke University Marine Laboratory, Beaufort, NC: *deadline February 10.*

. Fort Johnson Summer Undergraduate Research Program, College of Charleston, "Marine Organismal Health: Resilience and Response to Environmental Change"

. Georgia Tech, Aquatic Chemical Ecology (ACE): *applications open early December, due February 15.*

. Global Environmental Microbiology (GEM) Summer Course .

. Harvard University (Harvard Forest), Ecology.

. Indiana University, Center for the Integrative Study of Animal Behavior: *appplications due February 15.*

. Institute for Tropical Ecosystem Studies, Ecology and Evolution: *deadline February 28.*

- Kansas State University, Konza Prairie Biological Station: *applications due February 15.*

- W.K. Kellogg Biological Station, Michigan State University: *deadline March 1.*

- Michigan State University, Plant Genomics

- Michigan State University, Great Lakes Bioenergy Research Center.

- Mount Desert Island Biological Lab

- National Aeronautics and Space Administration (NASA) OSSI

- The Noble Foundation, Research Scholars in Plant Science

- Northwestern University and the Chicago Botanic Garden, plant biology and conservation

- Old Dominion University, Norfolk, Virginia.

- Ohio State, Stone Laboratory, Lake Erie, the oldest freshwater biological field station in the United States.

- Pepperdine University.

- Purdue University, West Lafayette, IN, SURF.

- Rocky Mountain Biological Laboratory.

- Shoals Marine Laboratory.

- Smithsonian Environmental Research Center.

- University of California, Santa Cruz, Doris Duke Conservation Scholars

- University of Delaware, College of Earth, Ocean, and Environment:

- University of Georgia, Fungal Genomics & Computational Biology:

- University of Maryland Center for Environmental Sciences Sea Grant's REU:

- University of Massachusetts, Boston, Intergrative and Evolutionary Biology-

- University of Michigan, School of Natural Resources and Environment, Doris Duke Conservation Scholars Program:

- University of North Carolina Charlotte, REU Summer Program Biology and Biotechnology:

- University of Nevada Las Vegas, Mechanisms of Evolution:

- University of Oregon, SPUR:

- University of Pittsburgh's TEC Program (Computational Biology):

- University of Virginia, Blandy Experimental Farm:

- University of Virginia, Mountain Lake Biological Station:

- University of Washington, Friday Harbor Laboratories:

• University of Wisconsin, Madison, Biological Interactions: Phenotype, Genotypre & Environment:

• Virginia Institute of Marine Science (VIMS):

• The Whitney Laboratory for Marine Bioscience:

• Woods Hole Oceanographic Institution:

• Woods Hole, The Polaris Project:

Programs Emphasizing Molecular Biology/Medicine

• Albert Einstein College of Medicine, SURP:

• Baylor College of Medicine, SMART Program:

• Boston University, Summer Institute in Biostatistics (SIBS)

• Brandeis University:

• Brigham and Women's STARS Program:

• Brigham and Women's Four Directions Summer Research Program (FDSRP):

• Broad Institute of MIT and Harvard- Summer Research Program (BSRP) Program:

• Burke Medical Research Institute:

• Centers for Disease Control and Prevention (CDC)-*various deadlines.*

- California Institute of Technology, SURF:

- Caltech, Amgen Scholars Program:

- Caltech, WAVE Fellows Program:

- Cold Spring Harbor: (includes Neuroscience):

- Colorado State University, Summer Program in Biochemistry & Molecular Biology:

- Columbia University, Barnard College, Amgen Scholars Program:

- Dana Farber/Harvard Cancer Center, CURE Program:

- Dartmouth, ASURE:

- Duke University:.

- Emory University, Natural and Biomedical Sciences:

- Fox Chase Cancer Center:

- Fred Hutchinson Cancer Research Center:

- Georgetown University ARCHES Fellowship:

- Gerstner Sloan Kettering:

- Harvard University, Summer Scholars Program-

- Harvard Medical School, Department of Cell Biology, Cell Biology Research Scholars Program (CRSP):.

- Harvard T.H. Chan School of Public Health, Multiple Summer Programs,: *Multiple opportunities*

- Howard Hughes Medical Institute-Janelia Farm Summer Program:

- The Jackson Laboratory:

- John Hopkins University- Visualization of Macromolecules in Biological Research:

- John Hopkins University, Institute for Nanobiotechnology:

- Joslin Diabetes Center:

- Maine Medical Center Research Institute (MMCRI):

- Mayo Clinic College of Medicine and Science Summer Undergraduate Research Fellowship (SURF):

- MDI Biological Laboratory

- Medical College of Wisconsin, SPUR:

- Medical University of South Carolina, DART Program:

- National Cancer Institute: *several opportunities, varying deadlines.*

- National Institute of Health:

- New York University, Sackler Institute:

- North Carolina State University, Summer Institute in Biostatistics:

- Ohio State University, Dept. of Molecular Genetics:

- Ohio University College of Osteopathic Medicine Summer Scholars:

- Oregon Health & Science University, Cell, Developmental and Cancer Biology

- Rockefeller University:

- Roswell Park Cancer Institute:

- Rutgers, RISE Program, (Piscataway, New Jersey):

- NeuroSURP, Rutgers,(Newark, New Jersey):

- Santa Fe Institute REU summer program:

- Scripps Research Institute, SURF Program, La Jolla, CA and Jupiter, FL:

- Stanford University, SSRP-Amgen:

- *Feb*SUNY Upstate Medical University, Syracuse.

- Texas A&M Health Science Center, College of Medicine

- Thomas Jefferson University College of Life Sciences:

- Tufts Sackler School of Graduate Biomedical Studies:

- University of Alabama at Birmingham, SIBS Program:

-

- University of Alabama at Birmingham, PARAdiGM Program:

- University of California at Berkeley, Amgen Scholars Program:

- University of California at San Francisco, SRTP:

- University of California at Los Angeles (UCLA)-Amgen Scholars Program:

- UCLA, B.I.G. Program:

- University of Cincinnati Medical School Summer Research Fellowship:

- University of Connecticut Health Center:

- University of Colorado Anshultz Medical Campus, Gates Center for Regenerative Medicine-

- University of Colorado, Colorado School of Public Health, Summer Institute of Biostatistics:

- University of Georgia, Microbiology:

- University of Iowa Summer Undergraduate MSTP program:

- University of Iowa, Microbiology:

- University of Iowa, College of Public Health, Summer Institute in Biostatistics:

- University of Massachusetts Medical School, Worcester, Massachusetts:

- University of Michigan, School of Public Health, The Future Public Health Leaders Program (FPHLP):

- University of Michigan Medical School: *Multiple opportunities & deadlines.*

- University of Minnesota, School of Public Health, Summer Institute in Biostatistics (SIBS):

- University of Minnesota-Life Sciences:

- University of Nebraska- Lincoln:

- University of Nebraska Medical Center:

- University of North Carolina – Chapel Hill:

- University of Oregon, REU in Molecular Biosciences: *no hard deadline, applications accepted on a rolling basis, offers of admission in late January, continuing until all slots are filled, usually by late March..*

- University of Pennsylvania ,TECBio: "Simulation and Visualization of Biological Systems at Multiple Scales":

- University of Pennsylvania, School of Medicine, Molecular Studies in Digestive and Liver Diseases:

- University of Pittsburgh School of Medicine Interdisciplinary Biomedical Sciences (SURP):

- University of Rochester, School of Medicine & Dentistry, Summer Scholars Program:

- University of Texas – Houston Health Sciences Center:

- University of Texas Southwestern Medical Center at Dallas:

- University of Virginia School of Medicine:

- University of Washington Neurological Surgery Summer Student Program:

- University of Wisconsin, Madison, Summer Research Opportunity Program (SROP):

- Vanderbilt University, Chemical Biology:

- Wadsworth Center, New York State Dept. of Health:

- Wake Forest School of Medicine, Summer Scholars Program:

- Washington University in St. Louis Amgen Scholars Program, BioMedRAP, and BP-ENDURE:

- Washington University in St. Louis Center for Engineering MechanoBiology (WU-CEMB)-

Programs Emphasizing Neuroscience

- Columbia University, The Summer of Translational Aging Research for Undergraduates (STAR U) Program:

- Huntington's Disease Society of America, Donald A. King HDSA Summer Research Fellowship:

- Orgeon Health & Science University Vollum/NGP Undergraduate Summer Research Program: .

- Oregon Health & Science University Neuroscience Postbaccalaureate Initiative: Biology Education

- Undergraduate Biology Education Research (UBER), University of Georgia:

- North Dakota State University Growing Up STEM Program:

- Rochester Institute of Technology, Discipline-Based Education Research (DBER), Model-based Reasoning in STEM Education:

- Teaching Experiences for Undergraduates (TEU):

- Washington State University Research in Interdisciplinary STEM Education (RISE) Program:

Internships in New York City

Columbia University Summer Undergraduate Research Fellowship (SURF) program. Only Columbia and Barnard undergraduates are eligible.

- Columbia University Amgen Scholars Program For Columbia/Barnard undergraduates as well as students from other U.S. universities. Columbia University NYSTEM Program For Columbia/Barnard undergraduates as well as students from other U.S. universities to perform stem cell research.

- Columbia University Chemistry research.
- Columbia University Center for Environmental Research & Conservation hosts the Summer Ecosystems Experiences for Undergraduates (SEE-U).
- Columbia University Lamont-Doherty Summer Internship Program for undergraduates.
- Columbia University Earth Intern Program for Columbia and Barnard Undergraduates.
- Albert Einstein College of Medicine. Biology.
- New York University- School of Medicine. Biomedical sciences.
- New York University – Center for Neural Science. Neuroscience.
- Rockefeller University. Biomedical sciences.
- Sloan Kettering Institute Biomedical sciences.
- Mount Sinai Graduate School of Biological Sciences. Biomedical sciences.
- Bronx Zoo Work with children in the zoo's camp program.
- Student Conservation Association Internships for college graduates in NY.
- Cold Spring Harbor Laboratories 10 week summer undergraduate research program (SURP).
- Irene and Eric Simon Brain Research Foundation Funding for a summer research internship in neuroscience.
- AHA Founders Affiliate Summer Student Fellowship 10 week research internship in cardiovascular research.

Biomedical laboratory research – elsewhere (Those limited to minorities are listed separately, below.)

- California Institute of Technology: Pasadena, CA. Amgen Scholars Program.
- Howard University: Washington, DC. Amgen Scholars

Program.

- Massachusetts   Institute   of Technology: Cambridge, MA. Amgen Scholars Program.
- Stanford University: Palo Alto, CA. Amgen Scholars Program.
- University of California: Berkeley, CA. Amgen Scholars Program.
- University of California: Los Angeles, CA. Amgen Scholars Program.
- University of California: San Diego, CA. Amgen Scholars Program.
- University of California: San Francisco, CA. Amgen Scholars Program.
- University of Washington: Seattle, WA. Amgen Scholars Program.
- Cold Spring Harbor Laboratory: Long Island, NY. Biology..
- UMDNJ – Graduate School of Biomedical Sciences: Stratford, NJ. Molecular/cellular biology.
- Brookhaven National Laboratory: Long Island, NY. Biology and chemistry.
- Rutgers University: Piscataway, NJ. Neuroscience.
- University of Connecticut Health Center: Quantitative cell biology.
- National Institute of Environmental Health Sciences: Research Triangle Park, NC.
- Emory University: Atlanta, GA.   All areas of biology, primate behavior.
- Children's Hospital Medical Center: Cincinnati, OH. Developmental biology.
- Loyola University – Stritch School of Medicine: Chicago IL. Microbiology and immunology.
- Indiana University: Bloomington IN.   Animal Behavior.
- Indiana University: Bloomington IN. Several pro-

grams.

- Mayo Clinic: Rochester, Minnesota. Biomedical sciences.
- University of Minnesota: St. Paul, MN. All areas of biology
- Washington University, St. Louis, MO. Biomedical Research Apprenticeship.
- Baylor College of Medicine: Houston, TX. All areas of biomedical sciences.
- University of Texas: Houston, TX. Summer Research Program
- University of Texas: San Antonio, TX. Biomedical lab research and clinical activity.
- University of Texas: Galveston, TX. Biomedical sciences.
- W.M. Keck Center for Computational Biology: Houston, TX. Computational biology.
- U.S. Department of Energy. Energy research undergraduate laboratory fellowship.
- Pasteur Foundation: Paris, France. Undergraduate Summer Internships at the Institut Pasteur
- Cornell Medical School: Gateways to the laboratory summer program
- Humboldt State University: 10-week Summer program in Ecology and Evolutionary Biology.
- Conservation International & University of Virginia: internship program
- UCSF: Nine week summer research 1ildlands1s1s in biological, biomedical, and behavioral sciences.
- Thomas Jefferson University: Summer undergraduate research program
- RISE (Research Internships in Science and Engineering): Undergraduate research in biology in Germany
- Northwestern University Institute for Nanotechnology: Summer internships in nanomedi-

cine and bionanotechnology

- Keck Graduate Institute: Claremont, CA. Summer REU Program in biotechnology & bioengineering.
- Virginia Tech: Bioengineering and Bioinformatics Summer Institute
- University of Chicago: 10 week summer research program at the Chicago Center for Systems Biology
- University of Texas Southwestern Medical Center: Summer fellowships in biological research
- AHA Founders Affiliate Summer Student Fellowship: 10 week research internship in cardiovascular research.
- University of Nebraska: Summer undergraduate research program

Ecology and environmental studies

- The Student Conservation Association
- Institute of Ecosystem Studies, Milbrook NY. Ecology.
- University of Colorado Boulder, CO. Behavior, ecology, evolution.
- Rocky Mountain Biological Laboratory, Crested Butte, CO. Field ecology..
- Point Reyes Bird Observatory, CA. Ornithology & field biology. No deadline, but best to apply early.
- Organization of Biological Field Stations. Lists field stations in US and overseas that are members of OBFS, many have summer programs (internships, courses, or volunteer work) in ecology and environmental studies.
- Smithsonian Environmental Research Center, Chesapeake Bay, MD. Environmental research and education.
- Environmental Careers Organization. Postings of nationwide internships in environmental fields.
- School for Field Studies. Summer internship after

completion of BA/BS degree.

- Operation Wallacea Biodiversity, forest biology, marine sciences in Indonesia.
- Mote Marine Laboratories Research experience for undergraduates (REU)
- ACEER Foundation. An exploration of plant based medicines from the Amazon and Andes.
- Woods Hole Oceanographic Institution. Summer student fellowships.
- SEE-U Black Rock Forest: 2.5 week long immersive introduction to ecology and field biology
- Steer – Center for Environmental Health Sciences

Marine biology – internships and courses

- Mote Marine Laboratory, Sarasota, FL. Estuarine science in Charlotte Harbor.
- Boston University/Marine Biological Laboratory, Woods Hole, MA. Coastal bays of New England.
- Woods Hole Oceanographic Institution, Woods Hole, MA. Marine biology.
- Marine Biological Laboratory, Summer 1ildlands1s. Woods Hole, MA. Marine biology.
- Marine Science Center (Northeastern U), Summer courses, near Boston.
- Shannon Point Marine Center, Puget Sound, WA. Marine sciences. Note additional Jan-June internship for minorities.
- Virginia Institute of Marine Science, Gloucester Point, VA. Marine biology.
- Mount Desert Island Biological Laboratory, ME. Marine biology.
- Center for Great Lakes Studies – UW-Milwaukee. Aquatic environments.
- Bermuda Biological Research Station. Marine biology courses and volunteer internships.
- Southampton College, Long Island, NY. Courses in

whale and dolphin behavior in Australia.
- Blakely Island Field Station, (Seattle Pacific University). Courses in marine biology and ecology.
- SeaCamp, Big Pine Key, FL. Staff/intern positions may be available.
- Whitney Laboratory Marine Biology at the U. Florida. Summer research internships in cell, molecular & neurobiology
- Marineland Dolphin Conservation Center Internships.
- Marine Biomedicine Sciences Center and Environmental Sciences Center. Summer fellowships for undergraduates in marine biology.

Other areas of biology

- Harvard Medical School. Undergraduate Summer Internship in Systems Biology
- Primate behavior. A listing of internships and volunteer positions, around the world.
- Hartford Hospital. Premed internship, clinical research and patient treatment.
- Summerbridge. Sites around the country, including Manhattan and Bronx. Get teaching experience.
- Advanced Studies Program – St. Paul's School, Concord, NH. Science teaching internship, field and lab work.
- National Museum of Natural History, Smithsonian Institution, Washington, DC. Systematics, evolution.
- University of Minnesota – Supercomputing Institute, Minneapolis, MN. Scientific computing, graphics and medicine.
- California Academy of Sciences, San Francisco, CA. Biological illustration.
- National Zoological Park, Washington DC. Zoo research. December deadline.
- Smithsonian InstitutionOther opportunities.
- National High Magnetic Field Laboratory Summer Re-

search Experiences for Undergraduates
- Urban Divers Estuary Conservancy Internships; clean and maintain NYCs waterways; summer and fall
- Astrobiology Summer Program at Penn State: 10 week internships for undergraduates.
- Computational & Systems Biology at Iowa State University: 8 week program for undergrads and first-year grad students
- GHEI Summer Serve & Learn: help the Ghana Health & Education Initiative implement its programs.
- University of Texas Southwestern Medical Center, 10 week summer internship in quantitative science and basic biomedical research
- Learn How to Become – Internships and career opportunities in the green sector

For students from disadvantaged backgrounds or minorities

- Summer Medical & Dental Education Program . free, six-week summer medical & dental school preparatory program
- National Institute of Health, Bethesda, MD. Undergraduate Scholarship Program
- New York University School of Medicine. Includes lab or clinical research.
- UNCF-MerckTwo summers of lab research at Merck, in Rhway, NJ or West Point PA, plus academic scholarship.
- University of Pennsylvania, School of Medicine. Pre-med enrichment program, includes lab or clinical research.
- BioMed RAPWashington University in St. Louis.
- University of Colorado, Boulder, CO. Molecular and organismal biology, genetics, biochemistry.
- Woods Hole Oceanographic Institution Minority Fellowships in Oceanography for Undergraduates

- Georgetown University **Gateway Exploration Program in Medicine for High School Students** https://som.georgetown.edu/diversityandinclusion/gep/
- **Georgetown University Summer Medical Institute & Medical Immersion Programs for High School Students** https://som.georgetown.edu/diversityandinclusion/internships/summer-medical-institute/
- **Georgetown University Mini Med School For High School Students** https://som.georgetown.edu/medicaleducation/specialprograms/minimed/
- Harvard Medical School, Boston, MA. Biomedical research.
- Harvard-MIT HST Summer Institute, Boston, MA. Biomedical optics or bioinformatics.
- Boston University, Boston, MA.
- Tufts University, Boston, MA.
- Caltech, Pasadena, CA. Biology, physics, math, earth sciences, chemistry.
- University of Oregon, Eugene, OR. Biology.
- Centers for Disease Control. Various programs, various deadlines.
- University of Pennsylvania, Center of Excellence on Minority Health. Pre-med enrichment, includes research.
- Leadership Alliance. Minority Internation Research Training Program.
- Washington University, St. Louis, MO. Biomedical Research Apprenticeship.
- Mit Summer Research Program (MSRP) Sophomores and Juniors interested in Science & Engineering
- Massachusetts Institute of Technology (MIT) MITES Program For High School Students
https://oeop.mit.edu/programs/mites/who-should-apply
- MURF Undergraduate Research Fellowship, Pasadena, CA. Ten-week summer research opportunity.
- NASA Science and Technology Institute Summer

Scholars: via UNCF Special Programs. Ten week program for undergrads in science, technology, engineering, and mathematics.

- NASA MUREP Minority University Research and Education Project Aerospace Academy (k-12) program offered at specific colleges and universities across the country
- Mentorship for Environmental Scholars: via UNCF Special Programs. 9 week paid internship; lab research in biotechnology, computer science, environmental science and engineering.
- MUST Program: via UNCF Special Programs. Awards scholarships and internships to undergraduate students pursuing Science, Technology, Engineering and Math degrees
- National Institute of Allergy and Infectious Diseases: research opportunities geared toward students with strong academic standing who are from populations underrepresented in biomedical research

Summer courses – Tuition is charged

- Columbia University – SEE-U. Summer Ecosystem Experience for Undergraduates, at Black Rock Forest, NY, Brazil.
- La Suerte and Ometepe Biological Field Stations, Costa Rica & Nicaragua. Variety of courses
- School for Field Studies. Hands-on environmental courses Canada, Australia, Costa Rica, Mexico, Kenya, West Indies.
- Institute for Field Education, Northwest Territories, Canada, Arctic field ecology.
- Wolf Park, Indiana. Wolf behavior, environmental education.
- Wildland Studies (San Francisco State U) Field explorations in remote environments to protect wildlife and 1ildlands.
- Health care delivery in the US and the

UK. England and Scotland.

- University of Pennsylvania School of Veterinary Medicine: VMD/Ph.D. program; biomedical research in zoonotic infectious diseases.
- Johns Hopkins University, Baltimore, MD. Tutoring, lab assistants in program for high school students.

Georgetown Summer Medical Institute (GSMI)

The summer program at Georgetown University School of Medicine offers outstanding medical course-based experiences for undergraduate and post-BACC students and remediating medical school students. All GSMI courses are taught by dedicated, internationally recognized professors from Georgetown University School of Medicine.

MEDICAL SCHOOLS OFFERING COMBINED BACCA-LAUREATE-MD PROGRAMS

ALABAMA University of Alabama School of Medicine

CALIFORNIA University of California, Riverside, School of Medicine

COLORADO University of Colorado School of Medicine

CONNECTICUT University of Connecticut School of Medicine

DISTRICT OF COLUMBIA The George Washington University School of Medicine and Health Sciences Howard University College of Medicine

FLORIDA Florida Atlantic University
Charles E. Schmidt College of Medicine
University of Central Florida College of Medicine
University of Florida College of Medicine
University of Miami Leonard M. Miller School of Medicine
University of South Florida Morsani College of Medicine

GEORGIA Medical College of Georgia at Augusta University

ILLINOIS Northwestern University Feinberg School of Medicine
University of Chicago Pritzker School of Medicine
University of Illinois College of Medicine

MASSACHUSETTS Boston University School of Medicine

MICHIGAN Wayne State University School of Medicine

MINNESOTA University of Minnesota Medical School

MISSOURI Saint Louis University School of Medicine
University of Missouri - Kansas City School of Medicine

NEVADA University of Nevada,
Reno, School of Medicine

NEW JERSEY Cooper Medical School of Rowan University
Rutgers New Jersey Medical School
Rutgers Robert Wood Johnson Medical School

NEW MEXICO University of New Mexico School of Medicine

NEW YORK Albany Medical College
CUNY School of Medicine
Donald and Barbara Zucker School of Medicine at Hofstra/Northwell
Renaissance School of Medicine at Stony Brook University
State University of New York Downstate Medical Center College of Medicine
State University of New York Upstate Medical University College of Medicine
University of Rochester School of Medicine and Dentistry

OHIO Case Western Reserve University School of Medicine
The University of Toledo College of Medicine and Life Sciences
University of Cincinnati College of Medicine

PENNSYLVANIA Drexel University College of Medicine
Lewis Katz School of Medicine at Temple University
Sidney Kimmel Medical College at Thomas Jefferson University
University of Pittsburgh School of Medicine

PUERTO RICO Ponce Health Sciences University School of Medicine

RHODE ISLAND Warren Alpert Medical School of Brown University

SOUTH CAROLINA University of South Carolina School of Medicine - Columbia

TENNESSEE Meharry Medical College School of Medicine

TEXAS Baylor College of Medicine
University of Texas Health Science Center at San Antonio Joe R. and Teresa Lozano Long School of Medicine
University of Texas Rio Grande Valley School of Medicine

VIRGINIA Eastern Virginia Medical School
Virginia Commonwealth University School of Medicine

WEST VIRGINIA Marshall University Joan C. Edwards School of Medicine

Reposted with permission from the AAMC

POST-BACCALAUREATE AND SMP PROGRAMS

Adelphi University Certificate in Basic Sciences for Health Professions

Agnes Scott College Post-Bacc Pre-Medical Program

American University Postbaccalaureate Premedical Certificate Program

Arizona State University Master of Science in the Science of Health Care Delivery
College of Health Solutions

Arizona State University Master of Science in Medical Nutrition

Avila University
Avila University Postbaccalaureate Program
Benedictine University Master of Science in Integrative Physiology
Bennington College Post Baccalaureate Premedical Program
Boston University Postbaccalaureate Certificate in Pre-Medical Studies
Boston University School of Medicine Master of Science in Medical Sciences Program
GMS, Boston Univ. School of Medicine

Boston University School of Medicine, Graduate Medical Sciences MS in Oral Health Sciences Program
Brandeis University Post-baccalaureate Premedical Program

Brown University, Warren Alpert Medical School Certificate in Medical Science
Brown University, Warren Alpert Medical School

Brown University, Warren Alpert Medical School Master of Science in Medical Sciences
Brown University, Warren Alpert Medical School

Bryn Mawr College Postbaccalaureate Premedical Program
Bryn Mawr College Canwyll House

California Northstate University (CNU)MPS to MD (2 + 4)-Combined Programs
California Northstate University

California Northstate University College of Health Sciences Pre-Med Post-Baccalaureate Plan
California State University, East Bay Post-Baccalaureate Pre-Professional Health Academic Program
California State University, Los Angeles Post-Baccalaureate Certificate Program for Pre-Health Professionals

California University of Science and Medicine Master of Biomedical Sciences Program

Campbell University Jerry M. Wallace School of Osteopathic Medicine (CUSOM)Master of Science in Biomedical Sciences (MSBS)

Carson-Newman University Postbaccalaureate Program

Case Western Reserve University Master of Science in Medical Physiology

Case Western Reserve University Master of Science in Applied Anatomy

Case Western Reserve University Master of Science in Pathology

Case Western Reserve University Master of Arts in Bioethics and Medical Humanities

Case Western Reserve University Master of Science in Nutrition

Case Western Reserve University Post-Baccalaureate Readiness Instruction for Medical Education (PRIME)
Cedars-Sinai Medical Center Master's Degree Program in Health Delivery Science (MHDS)

Chapman University Pre-Health Post-Baccalaureate Program

Charles R. Drew University of Medicine and Science CDU Enhanced Post Baccalaureate

Charles R. Drew University of Medicine and Science Graduate Biomedical Sciences (Master of Science)

Chatham University Master of Arts in Biomedical Studies (MABS)

Cleveland State University Post-Baccalaureate Program - Individualized Option

Cleveland State University and Northeast Ohio Medical University NEOMED-CSU Partnership for Urban Health Postbacc /M.D.

College of Science & Technology (CST); Temple University Basic Core in Health Sciences (BCHS) Post Baccalaureate Pre-Health Program

College of Science & Technology (CST): Temple University Advanced Core in Health Professions (ACHS) Post Baccalaureate Pre-Health Program

Colorado State University Master of Science in Biomedical Sciences (1 year)

Colorado State University Master of Science in Toxicology

Colorado State University Assisted Reproductive Technologies

Columbia University Postbaccalaureate Premedical Program

Columbia University Irving Medical Center Institute of Human Nutrition

Concordia College Post Baccalaureate Premedical Program

Cooper Medical School of Rowan University Advanced Premedical Studies Post Baccalaureate

Creighton University Creighton University Premedical Post baccalaureate

DePaul University Post-Baccalaureate Pre-Health Program

Des Moines University Master of Science in Anatomy

Des Moines University Master of Science in Biomedical Sciences Dominican University BMS, Post Baccalaureate Premedical Program

Drew University Pre-Medical Preparation Program

Drexel University College of Medicine Intensive Medical Sciences (IMS) Program

Drexel University College of Medicine Drexel Pathway to Medical School (DPMS) program

Drexel University College of Medicine Interdisciplinary Health Sciences (IHS) program

Drexel University College of Medicine Evening Post-Baccalaureate Pre-Medical (PMED) program

Drexel University College of Medicine Master of Biomedical Studies (MBS) Program

Drexel University College of Medicine Master of Medical Science (MMS) Program

Duke University School of Medicine Master of Biomedical Sciences

Duquesne University Duquesne University Post-Baccalaureate Pre-Medical and Health Professions Program

Eastern Mennonite University Gap Year Certificate

Eastern Mennonite University Biomedicine Certificate (1 year)

Eastern Mennonite University Master of Science in Premedicine (2 years)

Eastern Mennonite University Master of Science in Biomedicine (2 years)

Eastern Virginia Medical School Medical Master's Program (2-year option)

Eastern Virginia Medical School Medical Master's Program (1-year option)

Eastern Virginia Medical School Contemporary Human Anatomy Program (CHAP)

Elms College Postbaccalaureate Premedical Studies Certificate Program

Elms College Postbaccalaureate Premedical Program

Elms College Master of Biomedical Sciences Degree Program

Emory University Master of Arts in Bioethics

Farmingdale State College SUNY Certificate in the Sciences for Health Professions

Florida Atlantic University Post-Baccalaureate Medical Pathway Program

Florida International University Herbert Wertheim College of Medicine Graduate Certificate in Molecular and Biomedical Sciences

Florida State University College of Medicine Bridge to Clinical Medicine Program

Fordham University, Fordham School of Professional and Continuing Studies Fordham Post-Baccalaureate Pre-Medical/Pre-Health Program

Furman University Master of Science in Community Engaged Medicine

Geisel School of Medicine at Dartmouth The Dartmouth Institute for Health Policy and Clinical Practice

Geisinger Commonwealth School of Medicine Master of Biomedical Sciences

George Mason University/Georgetown University Advanced Biomedical Sciences Graduate Certificate Program

George Washington University George Washington University School of Medicine & Health Sciences: Masters in Anatomical & Translational Sciences

George Washington University GW Post-baccalaureate Premedicine Program

The George Washington University School of Medicine and Health Sciences

George Washington University School of Medicine and Health Sciences Graduate Certificate in Anatomical and Translational Sciences

George Squared George Squared Advanced Biomedical Sciences Graduate Certificate

Georgetown University MS Physiology & Biophysics - Complementary & Alternative Medicine (CAM) Program

Georgetown University Regular MS in Physiology

Georgetown University Special Master's Program - MS in Physiology

Georgetown University Post-Baccalaureate Pre-Medical Certificate Program

Georgetown University Master's in Systems Medicine

Georgetown University Georgetown Summer Medical Institute (GSMI)

Georgia State University Masters Degree in Biology Medical Science

Goucher College Post-Baccalaureate Premedical Program

Guilford College Post-Baccalaureate Pre-Medical and Pre-Health Studies

Hampton University Medical Science Masters Program
School of Science

Harvard Medical School Master of Medical Sciences in Immunology

Harvard University Division of Continuing Education Premedical Program

Heritage University Master of Arts in Medical Sciences

Hofstra University Premedical Post-Baccalaureate Certificate

Icahn School of Medicine at Mount Sinai Master of Science in Biomedical Sciences

Icahn School of Medicine at Mount Sinai Master of Science in Clinical Research

Icahn School of Medicine at Mount Sinai Clinical Research Training Program (Certificate)

Illinois Institute of Technology MS in Biology for the Health Professions

Indiana University Indiana University School of Medicine Master of Science Pre-Professional Degree Program

Indiana University School of Medicine Master of Science in Medical Science

Indiana University-Purdue University Indianapolis Pre-Professional Non-Thesis (PPNT) MS Program

Iowa State University 1-Year, Non-Thesis Master of Science in Biomedical Sciences

John Carroll University Pre-Medical Post-Baccalaureate Program

Johns Hopkins Bloomberg School of Public Health Master of Health Science, Environmental Health and Engineering

Johns Hopkins Bloomberg School of Public Health Master of Health Science (MHS) - Molecular

Johns Hopkins University Post-Baccalaureate Premedical Program

Johns Hopkins University Post-Baccalaureate Health Science Intensive Program
Center for Biotechnology Education

Johns Hopkins University Master of Health Science, Biochemistry and Molecular Biology, Bloomberg School of Public Health

Johnson & Wales University Pre-Medical & Pre-Health Professions Certificate

Kansas State University College of Veterinary Medicine One Year Master's in Biomedical Science

Keck Graduate Institute Post-Baccalaureate Premedical Certificate Program

Lake Erie College of Osteopathic Medicine Health Sciences Post Baccalaureate Program

Lake Erie College of Osteopathic Medicine, Bradenton Campus Masters of Medical Science

Larkin University Masters of Science in Biomedical Sciences

LaSalle University Postbaccalaureate Premedical Certificate Program

Lawrence Technological University Post-Baccalaureate Certificate in Premedical Studies

Lehigh University Healthcare Systems Engineering, MEng, Pre-Medical Post Baccalaureate

Lewis University B.S. Biomedical Sciences Program

Liberty University Master of Art In Medical Sciences

Liberty University School of Health Sciences Master of Science in Biomedical Sciences

Lipscomb University Master of Science in Biomolecular Science

Loras College Postbaccalaureate Pre-Medical/Pre-Health Program

Louisiana State University Shreveport Master of Science in Biological Sciences with a Health Sciences Concentration

Loyola Marymount University-Los Angeles LMU Pre-Medical/Pre-Dental Post-Baccalaureate Program

Loyola Marymount University, Seaver College of Science and Engineering (LMU Postbac)

Loyola University Chicago Master of Science in Medical Physiology

Loyola University Chicago MS in Infectious Disease and Immunology

LSU Health New Orleans School of Public Health Master of Public Health

Manhattanville College Post-Baccalaureate Pre-Health Professions (PBPH)

Marian University College of Osteopathic Medicine Master of Science in Biomedical Sciences

Marshall University Master of Science in Biomedical Sciences with an area of emphasis in Medical Sciences

Marymount Manhattan College Biology Post-Baccalaureate Program

Medical University of South Carolina Master of Science in Medical Sciences

Mercer University School of Medicine Master of Science in Preclinical Sciences

Mercer University School of Medicine Master of Science in Biomedical Sciences

Meredith College Pre-Health Post Baccalaureate Certificate Program

Michigan State University Medical Neuroscience

Midwestern University Master of Arts in Biomedical Science

Midwestern University Master of Arts in Biomedical Sciences

Midwestern University Master of Biomedical Sciences

Midwestern University Midwestern University: Master of Biomedical Sciences

Mills College Postbaccalaureate Program

Mississippi College Master's of Medical Sciences

Mississippi College Health Science Certificate Program

Montana State University Post Baccalaureate Pre-Medical Certificate

Montana State University Master of Science in Health Sciences

Morehouse School of Medicine Master of Science in Medical Sciences (MSMS) Degree

New York Medical College Basic Medical Sciences Interdisciplinary Program - Traditional Track
Graduate School of Basic Medical Sciences

New York Medical College Basic Medical Sciences Interdisciplinary Program - Accelerated Track Graduate School of Basic Medical Sciences

North Carolina State University Physiology Graduate Program

Northeastern State University Postbaccalaureate Prehealth Certificate Program

Northeastern University Post-Baccalaureate Pre-Medical

Northwest Native American Center of Excellence Wy'east Post-Baccalaureate Pathway
Robertson Life Sciences Building

Northwestern Health Sciences University Postbaccalaureate Pre-health

Northwestern University Program in Public Health

Northwestern University School of Professional Studies Professional Health Careers Premedicine Program

Nova Southeastern University MS, Biological Sciences with a concentration in Health Studies

NYU School of Medicine's Sackler Institute of Graduate Biomedical Sciences Master's in Biomedical Informatics

Oregon State University OSU Postbacc Premed Program

Ponce Health Sciences University - School of Medicine Master of Science in Medical Sciences

Providence College Pre-Health Professions Certificate Providence College School of Continuing Education

Purchase College SUNY Premedical Studies

Quinnipiac University Graduate Biomedical Sciences

Regis University Master of Science in Biomedical Sciences

Regis University Regis University - Biomedical Genetics and Genomics Graduate Certificate

Rider University Post-baccalaureate premedical studies

Rocky Vista University Master of Science in Biomedical Sciences (MSBS)

Rosalind Franklin University of Medicine & Science Master of Science in Biomedical Sciences

Rowan University Pre-Health Studies Post-Baccalaureate

Rush University MS in Biotechnology

Rutgers School of Graduate Studies New Brunswick-Piscataway Master of Biomedical Science

Rutgers School of Graduate Studies, Newark Health Science Campus Master's in Biomedical Sciences

Rutgers University New Brunswick Postbaccalaureate Prehealth Program

Saint Louis University Medical Anatomy & Physiology Certificate Program (MAPP)

Saint Xavier University Master of Science in Medical Science

Saint Xavier University Post Baccalaureate Certificate in Medical Science

Scripps College Post-Baccalaureate Premedical Program

Seattle University Postbaccalaureate Premedical Program

Shoreline Community College Post Baccalaureate Studies for the Health Professions

South Dakota State University Human Biology

SUNY College at Old Westbury Post-baccalaureate Premedical Studies

SUNY Upstate Medical University Med Prep Academic Enhancement MS in Medical Technology

Syracuse University M.S. in Biomedical Forensic Sciences Forensic & National Security Sciences Institute

Temple University School of Medicine Basic Core In Medical Science (BCMS) Post Baccalaureate PreMedical Program

Temple University School of Medicine Advanced Core in Medical Science Post Baccalaureate PreMedical Program
Texas Tech University Health Sciences Center Graduate Medical Sciences, M.S. in Biomedical Sciences

The City College of New York The Program In Pre-Medical Studies Accelerated Post-Baccalaureate Certificate in Health Professions Preparation

The City College of New York The City College of New York Post-Baccalaureate Program

The George Washington University MSHS in Medical Laboratory Science

The George Washington University Post Baccalaureate Certificate in Blood Banking

The George Washington University MSHS in Laboratory Medicine Program

The George Washington University MSHS in Immunohematology and Biotechnology

The George Washington University Post Baccalaureate Certificate in Clinical Chemistry

The George Washington University Post Baccalaureate Certificate in Hematology

The George Washington University MSHS in Translational Microbiology

The George Washington University Post Baccalaureate Certificate in Microbiology

The George Washington University Post Baccalaureate Certificate in Medical Laboratory Science

The George Washington University Post-baccalaureate Certificate in Molecular Diagnostic Sciences

The George Washington University MSHS in Molecular Diagnostic Sciences

The George Washington University MSHS in Clinical Microbiology

The Ohio State University MEDPATH Post Baccalaureate Program

Thomas Jefferson University Postbaccalaureate Pre-Professional Program (P4)

Touro College of Osteopathic Medicine MS in Interdisciplinary Studies in Biological and Physical Sciences

Tufts University Post Baccalaureate Premedical Program

Tufts University School of Medicine MS in Biomedical Sciences

Tulane University Cell and Molecular Biology One Year Masters

Tulane University School of Medicine One Year Master's in Medical Genetics and Genomics

Tulane University School of Medicine One-Year Masters Program in Microbiology and Immunology

Tulane University School of Medicine One Year Master's in Pharmacology Program

Tulane University School of Medicine One Year Master's Program in Physiology

Tulane University School of Medicine Structural & Cellular Biology-Anatomy Certification & Leadership Program

Tulane University School of Medicine Structural & Cellular Biology ~ Masters Degree Program ~ MS Anatomy

Tulane University School of Medicine One Year Master of Science in Molecular Medicine

Tulane University School of Medicine Two Year Master of Science in Molecular and Cellular Pathobiology

Tulane University School of Medicine One-Year Masters Program in Biochemistry & Molecular Biology

UC Berkeley Extension Post-Baccalaureate Health Professions Certificate Program

UC Davis UC Davis Health Professions Post-Baccalaureate Program

UC Davis School of Medicine Postbaccalaureate Program

UC Irvine School of Medicine UC Irvine School of Medicine Post-baccalaureate Program

UC San Diego UC San Diego Post Baccalaureate Premedical Program

UCLA Extension Pre-Medical and General Science Studies Certificate

UCSF Master of Science in Biomedical Imaging (MSBI) Graduate Program

UMKC College of Arts and Sciences Pre-Health Program

University at Buffalo, State University of New York Natural Sciences Interdisciplinary MS
Jacobs School of Medicine and Biomedical Sciences

University at Buffalo, The State University of New York Special Master's Program (SMP) in Biological Sciences

University of Alabama at Birmingham Master of Science Biomedical and Health Science

University of California, Irvine UCI School Postbaccalaureate Premedical Program
UCI School Postbaccalaureate Premedical Program

University of California, San Francisco UCSF Interprofessional Health Post Baccalaureate Program

University of Cincinnati College of Medicine Special Master's Program in Physiology

University of Cincinnati, College of Medicine Master's in Pharmacology with emphasis on Preclinical & Clinical Drug Safety
Department of Pharmacology & Systems Physiology

University of Colorado Anschutz Medical Campus Master of Science in Modern Human Anatomy

University of Colorado Boulder Post Baccalaureate Health Professions Program for Career Changers (Med, Dent, Vet, PT, PA, etc.)

University of Colorado Boulder University of Colorado Boulder: Flexible Post-Baccalaureate Option

University of Connecticut Medicine and Dental Medicine Post-Baccalaureate Program

University of Delaware Premedical Post Baccalaureate Certificate Program
Center for Health Profession Studies

University of Denver Professional Science Master's in Biomedical Science

University of Florida Pre-Health Post-Baccalaureate Program (PHPB)

University of Hawaii John A. Burns School of Medicine'Imi Ho'ōla Post-Baccalaureate Program

University of Illinois Medical College Master of Science in Medical Physiology

University of Kentucky Master of Science in Medical Sciences

University of Louisville Postbaccalaureate Pre-medical Program
College of A & S Advising PBPMP Gardiner Hall

University of Louisville Master of Science in Physiology
Department of Physiology

University of Maryland Science in the Evening

University of Miami Pre-Health Post-Baccalaureate Program

University of Michigan Medical School M.S. Program in Physiology

University of Michigan Medical School, Office of Graduate & Postdoctoral Studies (OGPS)Postbac MEDPREP Program: Post-

Baccalaureate Premedical Program

University of North Carolina at Greensboro Post-Baccalaureate Pre-Professional Program
Post-Baccalaureate Pre-Professional Program, UNC-Greensboro

University of North Texas Health Science Center Biomedical Science Graduate Program

University of Northern Colorado Master's in Biomedical Science Online

University of Northern Colorado Online Master's in Biology, non-thesis

University of Pennsylvania Pre-Health Programs

University of Pittsburgh Biomedical Masters Program

University of Rochester Post-baccalaureate Pre-Health Program

University of South Florida Morsani College of Medicine Masters in Medical Science with a Concentration in Interdisciplinary Medical Science (IMS)

University of Southern California USC Postbaccalaureate Premedical Program

University of Toledo Master of Science in Biomedical Science in Medical Sciences (MSBS-MS)

University of Virginia U.Va. Post-Baccalaureate Pre-Medical Program

Vanderbilt University Master's Program in Biomedical Sciences
Master's Program In Biomedical Sciences

Virginia Commonwealth University PreMedical Graduate Certificate Program (CERT)

Wake Forest University Graduate School of Arts and Sciences, Biomedical Programs Biomedical Sciences Pre-health Master of Science

Wayne State University PreMedical Post Baccalaureate Program

West Virginia University Master of Science in the Health Sciences

MD/PHD PROGRAMS

Alabama

University of Alabama School of Medicine Birmingham, Ala.

University of South Alabama College of Medicine Mobile, Ala.

Arizona

University of Arizona College of Medicine Tucson, Ariz.

University of Arizona College of Medicine - Phoenix Phoenix, Ariz.

Arkansas

University of Arkansas College of Medicine Little Rock, Ark.

California

Loma Linda University School of Medicine Loma Linda, Calif.

Stanford University School of Medicine Stanford, Calif.

University of California, Davis School of Medicine Davis, Calif.

University of California, Irvine School of Medicine Irvine, Calif.

University of California, Los Angeles School of Medicine Los Angeles, Calif.

University of California, San Diego School of Medicine La Jolla, Calif.

University of California, San Francisco School of Medicine San Francisco, Calif.

Keck School of Medicine of the University of Southern California Los Angeles, Calif.

Colorado

University of Colorado Health Sciences Center Denver, Colo.

Connecticut

University of Connecticut School of Medicine Farmington, Conn.

Yale University School of Medicine New Haven, Conn.

District of Columbia

Georgetown University School of Medicine Washington, D.C.

Howard University College of Medicine Washington, D.C.

Florida

University of Florida College of Medicine Gainesville, Fla.

University of Miami Miller School of Medicine Miami, Fla.

University of South Florida College of Medicine Tampa, Fla.

Georgia

Emory University School of Medicine Atlanta, Ga.

Medical College of Georgia Augusta, Ga.

Morehouse School of Medicine Atlanta, Ga.

Medical College of Georgia at Augusta University Augusta, Ga.

Illinois

Loyola University of Chicago - Stritch School of Medicine Maywood, Ill.

Northwestern University Medical School Chicago, Ill.

Rosalind Franklin University of Medicine and Science - Chicago Medical School North Chicago, Ill.

University of Chicago Pritzker School of Medicine (MTSP) Chicago, Ill.

University of Chicago Pritzker School of Medicine (MD/PhD) Chicago, Ill.

University of Illinois at Chicago College of Medicine Chicago, Ill.

University of Illinois at Urbana-Champaign College of Medicine Urbana, Ill.

Indiana

Indiana University School of Medicine Indianapolis, Ind.

Iowa

University of Iowa College of Medicine Iowa City, Iowa

Kansas

University of Kansas School of Medicine Kansas City, Kan.

Kentucky

University of Kentucky College of Medicine Lexington, Ky.

University of Louisville School of Medicine Louisville, Ky.

Louisiana

Louisiana State University, New Orleans School of Medicine New Orleans, La.

Louisiana State University, Shreveport School of Medicine Shreveport, La.

Tulane University School of Medicine New Orleans, La.

Maryland

Johns Hopkins University School of Medicine Baltimore, Md.

National Institutes of Health Intramural MD-PhD Partnership Bethesda, Md.

Uniformed Services University of the Health Sciences Bethesda, Md.

University of Maryland at Baltimore School of Medicine Baltimore, Md.

Massachusetts

Boston University School of Medicine Boston, Mass.

Harvard Medical School Boston, Mass.

Tufts University School of Medicine Boston, Mass.

University of Massachusetts Medical School Worcester, Mass.

Michigan

Michigan State University College of Medicine East Lansing, Mich.

University of Michigan Medical School Ann Arbor, Mich.

Wayne State University School of Medicine Detroit, Mich.

Minnesota

Mayo Medical School Rochester, Minn.

University of Minnesota Medical School Minneapolis, Minn.

Mississippi

University of Mississippi School of Medicine Jackson, Miss.

Missouri

Saint Louis University School of Medicine St. Louis, Mo.

University of Missouri - Columbia School of Medicine Columbia, Mo.

University of Missouri - Kansas City School of Medicine Kansas City, Mo.

Washington University School of Medicine St. Louis, Mo.

Nebraska

Creighton University School of Medicine Omaha, Neb.

University of Nebraska College of Medicine Omaha, Neb.

Nevada

University of Nevada School of Medicine Reno, Nev.

New Hampshire

Geisel School of Medicine at Dartmouth Hanover, N.H.

New Jersey

University of Medicine & Dentistry of New Jersey - New Jersey Medical School Newark, N.J.

University of Medicine & Dentistry of New Jersey - Robert Wood Johnson Medical School Piscataway, N.J.

New Mexico

University of New Mexico School of Medicine Albuquerque, N.M.

New York

Albany Medical College Albany, N.Y.

Albert Einstein College of Medicine of Yeshiva University Bronx, N.Y.

Columbia University College of Physicians and Surgeons New York, N.Y.

Hofstra North Shore - LIJ School of Medicine Hempstead, N.Y.

Weill Cornell/Rockefeller/Sloan-Kettering Tri-Institutional MD/PhD

Program New York, N.Y.

Mount Sinai School of Medicine New York, N.Y.

New York Medical College Valhalla, N.Y.

New York University School of Medicine New York, N.Y.

SUNY at Buffalo School of Medicine Buffalo, N.Y.

SUNY at Stony Brook Health Sciences Center Stony Brook, N.Y.

SUNY Downstate Medical Center College of Medicine Brooklyn, N.Y.

SUNY Upstate Medical University Syracuse, N.Y.

University of Rochester School of Medicine Rochester, N.Y.

North Carolina

Wake Forest School of Medicine Winston-Salem, N.C.

Brody School of Medicine at East Carolina University Greenville, N.C.

Duke University School of Medicine Durham, N.C.

University of North Carolina at Chapel Hill School of Medicine Chapel Hill, N.C.

North Dakota

University of North Dakota School of Medicine Grand Forks, N.D.

Ohio

Case Western Reserve University School of Medicine Cleveland, Ohio

Northeastern Ohio College of Medicine Rootstown, Ohio

Ohio State University College of Medicine Columbus, Ohio

University of Cincinnati College of Medicine Cincinnati, Ohio

University of Toledo College of Medicine Toledo, Ohio

Wright State University School of Medicine Dayton, Ohio

Oklahoma

University of Oklahoma Health Sciences Center Oklahoma City, Okla.

Oregon

Oregon Health Sciences University School of Medicine Portland, Ore.

Pennsylvania

Drexel University College of Medicine Philadelphia, Pa.

Sidney Kimmel Medical College at Thomas Jefferson University Philadelphia, Pa.

Penn State University College of Medicine Hershey, Pa.

University of Pennsylvania School of Medicine Philadelphia, Pa.

University of Pittsburgh School of Medicine Pittsburgh, Pa.

Temple University School of Medicine Philadelphia, Pa.

Rhode Island

Brown University School of Medicine Providence, R.I.

South Carolina

Medical University of South Carolina Charleston, S.C.

University of South Carolina School of Medicine Columbia, S.C.

South Dakota

University of South Dakota School of Medicine Vermillion, S.D.

Tennessee

East Tennessee State University James H. Quillen College of Medicine Johnson City, Tenn.

Meharry Medical College School of Medicine Nashville, Tenn.

University of Tennessee, Memphis College of Medicine Memphis, Tenn.

Vanderbilt University School of Medicine Nashville, Tenn.

Texas

Baylor College of Medicine Houston, Texas

McGovern Medical School at UTHealth/MD Anderson Cancer Center/ University of Puerto Rico Tri-Institutional Program Houston, Texas

Texas A&M University Health Sciences Center College of Medicine College Station, Texas

Texas Tech University School of Medicine Lubbock, Texas

University of Texas at Austin Austin, Texas

University of Texas Medical Branch at Galveston Galveston, Texas

University of Texas, San Antonio Medical School San Antonio, Texas

University of Texas, Southwestern Med Center - Dallas Dallas, Texas

Utah

University of Utah School of Medicine Salt Lake City, Utah

Vermont

University of Vermont College of Medicine Burlington, Vt.

Virginia

Eastern Virginia Medical School Norfolk, Va.

Virginia Commonwealth University School of Medicine Richmond, Va.

University of Virginia School of Medicine Charlottesville, Va.

Washington

University of Washington School of Medicine Seattle, Wash.

West Virginia

Marshall University School of Medicine Huntington, W.Va.

West Virginia University School of Medicine Morgantown, W.Va.

Wisconsin

Medical College of Wisconsin Milwaukee, Wisc.

University of Wisconsin Medical School Madison, Wisc.

Canada

McGill University Faculty of Medicine Montreal, Quebec

McMaster University of Faculty of Health Sciences Hamilton, Ontario

Memorial University of Newfoundland Faculty of Medicine St. John's, Newfoundland and Labrador

Universite de Montreal Faculte de Medecine Montreal, Quebec

Universite de Sherbrooke Faculte de Medecine Sherbrooke, Quebec

Universite Laval Faculte de Medecine Quebec, Quebec

University of Alberta Faculty of Medicine and Dentistry Edmonton,

Alberta

University of Calgary Faculty of Medicine Calgary, Alberta

University of British Columbia Faculty of Medicine Vancouver, British Columbia

University of Manitoba Faculty of Medicine Winnipeg, Manitoba

University of Saskatchewan College of Medicine Saskatoon, Saskatchewan

University of Toronto Faculty of Medicine Toronto, Ontario

University of Western Ontario London, Ontario

Related Programs

NIH MD-PhD Partnership Program

Source: AAMC

www.ingramcontent.com/pod-product-compliance
Lightning Source LLC
LaVergne TN
LVHW051059080426
835508LV00019B/1971